Challenging Cases in Spine Surgery

Thieme

Challenging Cases in Spine Surgery

Muwaffak Abdulhak, M.D.
Director
Complex Spine Surgery Program
Department of Neurosurgery
Henry Ford Hospital
Detroit, Michigan

Shaden Marzouk, M.D.
Spine Fellow
Department of Neurosurgery
Northwestern Memorial Hospital
Chicago, Illinois

Thieme
New York • Stuttgart

Thieme Medical Publishers, Inc.
333 Seventh Ave.
New York, NY 10001

Editor: Tim Hiscock
Vice-President, Production and Electronic Publishing: Anne T. Vinnicombe
Production Editor: Becky Dille
Sales Director: Ross Lumpkin
Associate Marketing Director: Verena Diem
Chief Financial Officer: Peter van Woerden
President: Brian D. Scanlan
Compositor: Alden Books
Printer: Maple-Vail Book Manufacturing Group

Library of Congress Cataloging-in-Publication Data

Abdulhak, Muwaffak.
Challenging cases in spine surgery / Muwaffak Abdulhak, Shaden Marzouk.
p ; cm.
Includes bibliographical references and index.
ISBN 1-58890-393-1 (TMP : alk. paper) – ISBN 3-13-141941-5 (GTV : alk. paper)
1. Spine–Surgery. 2. Spine–Surgery–Miscellanea. I. Marzouk, Shaden. II. Title
DNLM: 1. Spinal Diseases–surgery–Case Reports. 2. Neurosurgical Procedures–methods–Case Reports. WE 725 A136c
20061
RD768TA23 2006
617 5 6059–dc22 2005021935

Important note: Medical knowledge is ever-changing. As new research and clinical experience broaden our knowledge, changes in treatment and drug therapy may be required. The authors and editors of the material herein have consulted sources believed to be reliable in their efforts to provide information that is complete and in accord with the standards accepted at the time of publication. However, in the view of the possibility of human error by the authors, editors, or publisher of the work herein or changes in medical knowledge, neither the authors, editors, or publisher, nor any other party who has been involved in the preparation of this work, warrants that the information contained herein is in every respect accurate or complete, and they are not responsible for any errors or omissions or for the results obtained from use of such information. Readers are encouraged to confirm the information contained herein with other sources. For example, readers are advised to check the product information sheet included in the package of each drug they plan to administer to be certain that the information contained in this publication is accurate and that changes have not been made in the recommended dose or in the contraindications for administration. This recommendation is of particular importance in connection with new or infrequently used drugs.

Printed in the United States of America

5 4 3 2 1

TMP ISBN 1-58890-393-1
GTV ISBN 3 13 141941 5

Contents

PART V INFECTION

PART VI CONGENITAL

Preface

Spine surgery is a multidisciplinary specialty, with cases encompassing the spectrum of complexity. New technologies are always being introduced, and while one makes decisions based on a clinical picture, the importance of radiologic findings cannot be discounted. Whether you are a surgeon, pain management or rehabilitation specialist, primary care doctor, radiologist, or physician treating spine patients, your world is evolving. Whether you are a student of these subspecialties or a veteran practitioner, you will encounter cases that stretch your clinical acumen. In our center, we have experienced the gamut of complex spine surgery cases, and we discuss them in this book, specifically the radiologic and pathologic findings, treatment, rationale, and key points. Up-to-date technologies, such as bone morphogenetic protein and percutaneous spine surgery, are discussed. Pathognomonic magnetic resonance imaging scans, computed tomography scans, myelograms, angiograms, plain x-rays, and pathology slides supplement the text. The focus is the thought process and reasoning that accompanies the management of these cases from clinical presentation, to classic radiology findings, to operative versus conservative treatments.

Through a case study format, various points in treating spine patients are emphasized. Suggested readings are provided at the end of each case. Management of challenging traumatic, inflammatory, degenerative, neoplastic, infectious, and congenital spine cases are covered. It is our hope that this book will satisfy the needs of the busy practitioner for concise, to-the-point information as well as the student looking for more detail.

Acknowledgments

This project would not have been possible without the contributions of many people. We wish to thank our department for their support, and, in particular, our chairman Dr. Mark Rosenblum for his encouragement and academic leadership. We would also like to thank the spine team for these cases, and especially Jennifer Tribu, R.N. Our appreciation goes to Dr. Khang-Loon Ho, who provided invaluable assistance with the pathology figures, and to our in-house medical photography team, especially Ray Manning and Patricia Maldoon for their efficiency. Jennifer Burch and Shree Venkat, third-year medical students at Wayne State University Medical School, deserve a special acknowledgment for their help with preparatory work.

No words of gratitude would be complete without mentioning our families. Their support and willingness to endure of our long working hours makes this all worthwhile. Thank you to Nuha, Yamar, and Sinan Abdulhak, and Mohamed, Hanar, and Youssef Marzouk.

To our families

■ PART I ■

Trauma

1

Odontoid Fracture Type I

■ Presentation

A 19-year-old woman was in a motor vehicle accident. She was neurologically intact, but had some neck pain.

■ Radiologic Findings

A sagittal reconstructed cervical computed tomography (CT) scan displays a displaced fracture through the tip of the odontoid (**Fig. 1–1**).

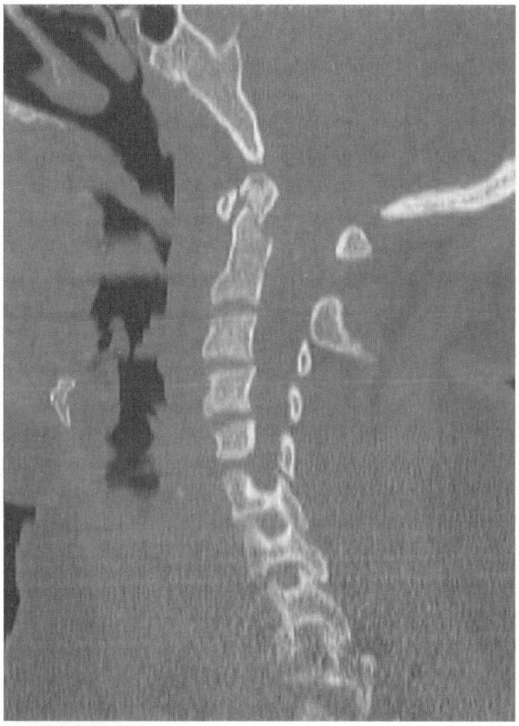

FIGURE 1–1 Type I odontoid fracture as seen on sagittal reconstructed CT.

■ Diagnosis

Type I odontoid fracture

■ Treatment

As presented on a lateral cervical x-ray, reduction and fixation with an odontoid screw was accomplished (**Fig. 1–2**).

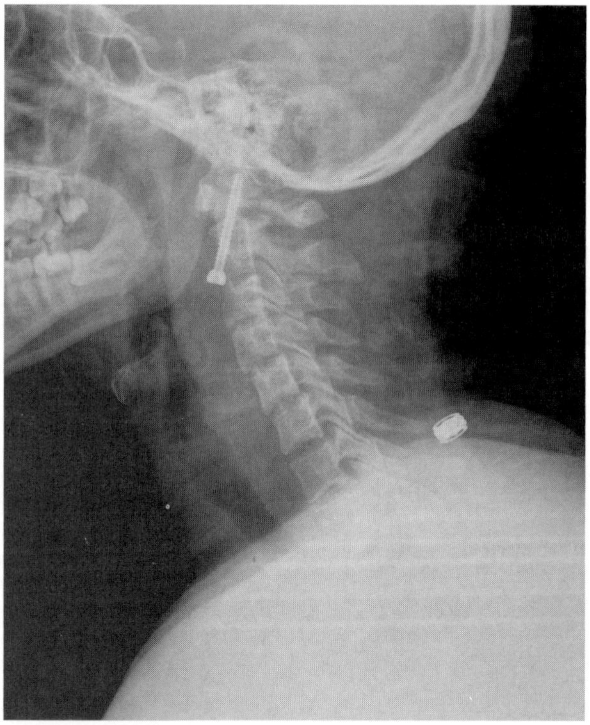

FIGURE 1–2 Postoperative x-ray.

■ Discussion

A type I odontoid fracture is a rare avulsion injury through the tip of the dens cephalad to the transverse ligament. It usually results from severe rotational and lateral bending forces, causing unilateral avulsion of the bone through the alar and apical ligaments. It is generally categorized as a stable injury, although association with occipitocervical dislocation has been reported. When the latter is ruled out, treatment is typically an external orthosis.

Os odontoideum is frequently confused with the above entity. Os odontoideum represents a round, smooth ossicle, with a definite gap between the os and the dens, lying above the level of the superior articular facet. The precipitating factor is debatable but thought to be mostly congenital. It is seen in the following syndromes: Klippel-Feil, myelodysplasia, epiphyseal dysplasia, and Down syndrome. Posttraumatic causes of os odontoideum have also been reported. It is associated with a higher incidence of occipitocervical dislocation.

This patient refused to wear an external orthosis. With her degree of fracture displacement, that noncompliance was concerning. Her anterolisthesis was reduced intraoperatively under fluoroscopy, and then fixated with an odontoid screw. Postoperatively she recovered without sequelae.

SUGGESTED READING

Greene KA, Dickman CA, Marciano FF, Drabier JB, Hadley MNB, Sonntag VK. Acute axis fractures: analysis of management and outcome in 340 consecutive cases. Spine 1997;22:1843–1852

2

Transodontoid Screw for Type II Odontoid Fracture

■ Presentation

A 63-year-old woman fell while riding a bike. She sustained a type II odontoid fracture and was initially treated with halo immobilization for 6 weeks. On follow-up x-ray, she continued to have subluxation but remained neurologically intact.

■ Radiologic Findings

Computed tomography (CT) reconstruction of the C-spine (**Fig. 2–1**) is notable for a type II odontoid fracture with severe subluxation of over 10 mm.

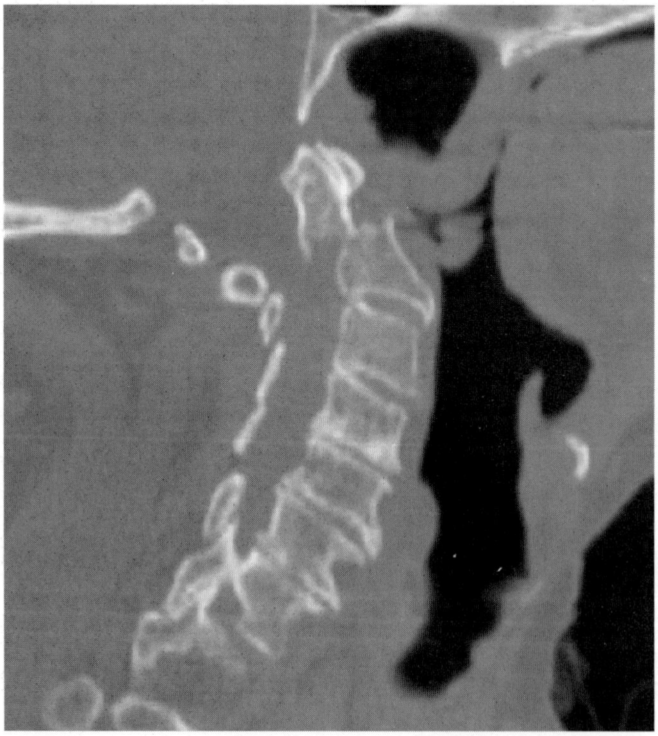

FIGURE 2–1 Reconstructed CT of the C-spine shows a prominent subluxation between the fracture fragment and body of the dens.

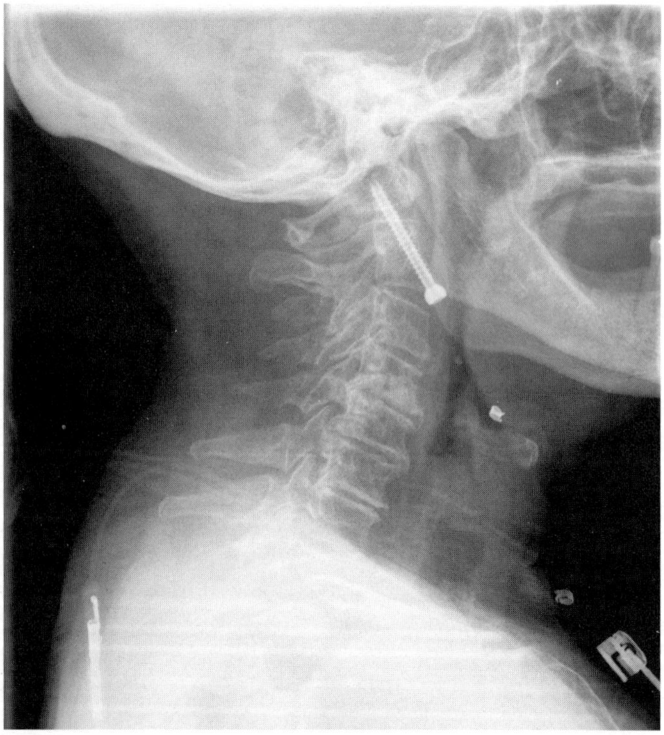

FIGURE 2–2 Postoperative x-ray with odontoid screw in place.

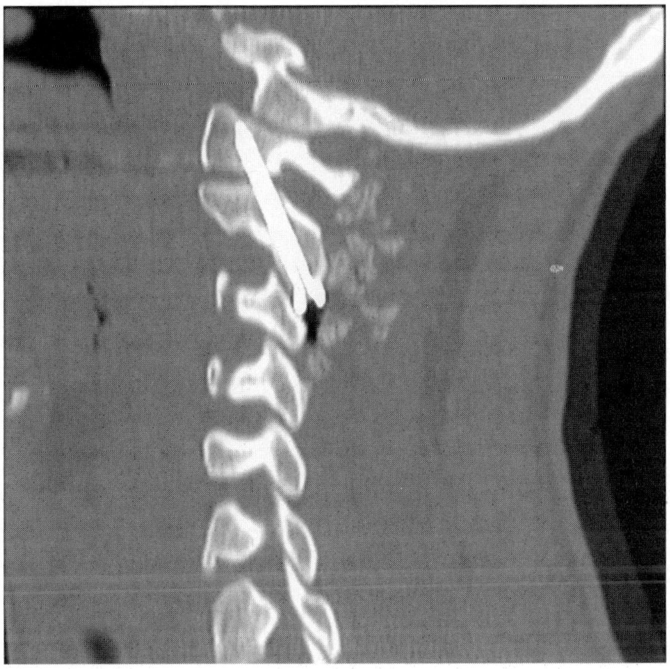

FIGURE 4–3 Computed tomography reconstruction with transarticular screw displayed.

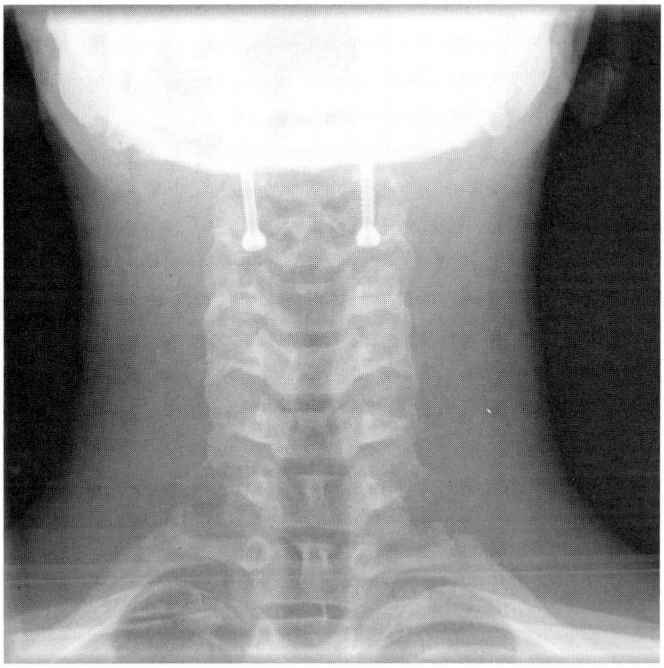

FIGURE 4–4 Postoperative AP cervical x-ray with screws displayed.

■ Diagnosis

Atlantoaxial instability

■ Treatment

Transarticular screws were placed (**Figs. 4–3** and **4–4**).

■ Discussion

The causes of atlantoaxial instability include trauma, congenital abnormality, rheumatoid arthritis, or iatrogenic injury. A series of ligaments hold together the occipitoatlantoaxial joint, such as the apical, alar, transverse, anterior, and posterior atlanto-occipital and tectoral membranes. The most important of these is the transverse ligament. An overhang of 6.9 mm or more of the C1 on 2 lateral masses on anteroposterior (AP) imaging of the cervical spine indicates an incompetent transverse ligament.

The distance between the odontoid and the posterior border of the anterior arch of the atlas is called the atlantodental interval (ADI). Instability is present if this measurement is greater than 3 mm in adults and 5 mm in children. Although there is greater room for the spinal cord at this level, neurologic deficit can occur. Also, isolated neck pain can occur. At diagnosis the neck should be protected with a rigid orthosis, and surgery is needed for cases with ligamentous instability.

Transarticular screws have been shown to provide a more solid fusion than posterior wiring techniques. An immediate, rigid three-column fixation with direct facet arthrodesis is achieved. This technique is viable for traumatic or inflammatory atlantoaxial instability, or for C2 pseudoarthrosis. Contraindications are an aberrant vertebral artery, inability to sufficiently align C1 and C2, or poor bone quality. This surgery is performed with biplanar fluoroscopy and neurophysiologic monitoring.

SUGGESTED READINGS

Spence KF Jr, Decker S, Sell KW. Bursting atlantal fracture associated with rupture of the transverse ligament. J Bone Joint Surg Am 1970;52:543–549

Taggard DA, Kraut MA, Clark CR, Traynelis VC. Case control study comparing the efficacy of surgical techniques for C1–2 arthrodesis. J Spinal Disord Tech 2004;17:189–194

5

Bilateral Locked Facets

■ Presentation

A 51-year-old woman was assaulted during a bar fight and became a C5 quadriplegic.

■ Radiologic Findings

Axial CT through the area of injury demonstrates inversion of the normal appearance of the facets—"naked facets" (**Fig. 5–1**). The C5 inferior facet is located anterior to the C6 superior facet, indicating bilaterally jumped and locked facets. This also indicates an anterolisthesis of 50% or greater.

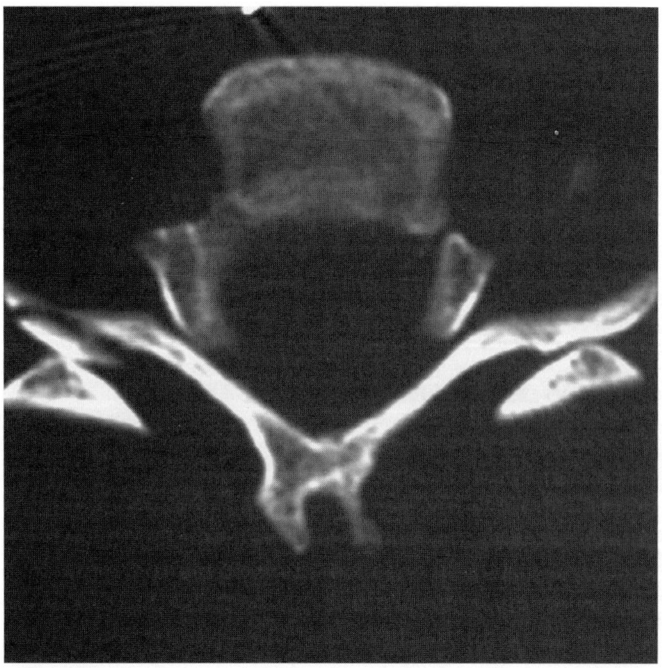

FIGURE 5–1 Axial computed tomography (CT) showing the "reversal hamburger" sign. The orientation of the facets is reversed because C5 is anterolisthesed on C6.

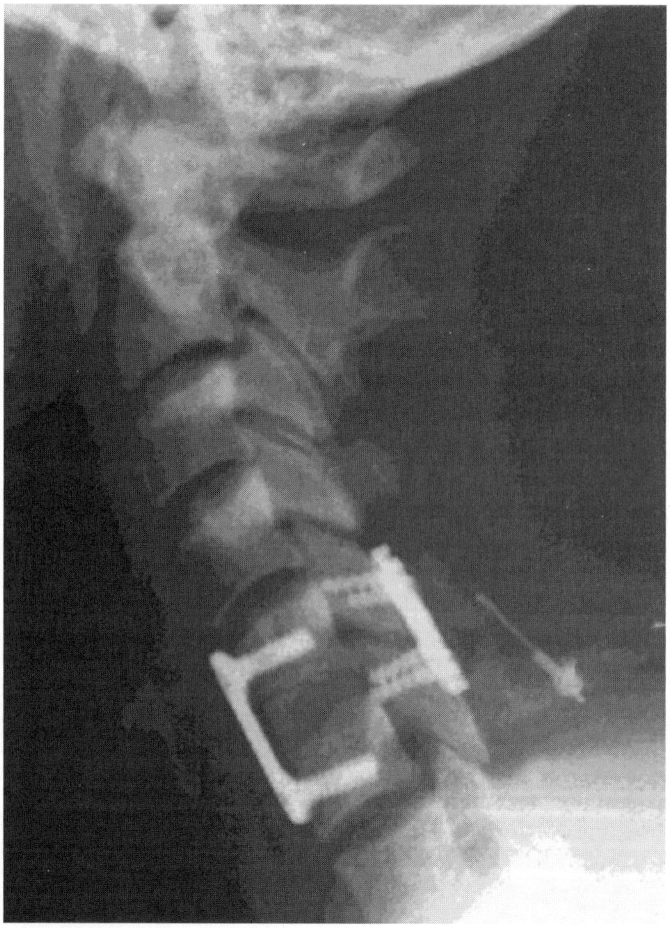

FIGURE 5–2 Postoperative lateral C-spine x-ray displaying a 360-degree fusion construct from the patient in **Fig. 5–1**.

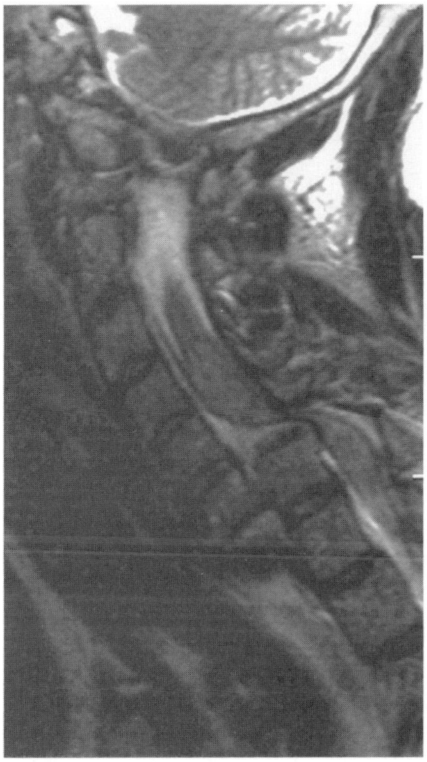

FIGURE 5–3 Preoperative spondyloptosis.

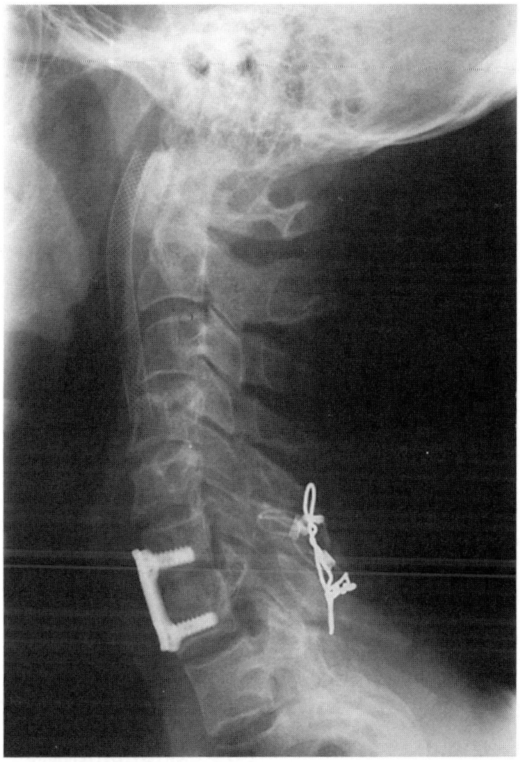

FIGURE 5–4 Postoperative correction of the spondyloptosis patient.

■ Diagnosis

Traumatic spondylolisthesis with cervical cord injury

■ Treatment

A 360-degree fusion was done (**Fig. 5–2**).

■ Discussion

Bilaterally dislocated facets are a grossly unstable cervical spine injury resulting from severe trauma to the spine. This is a three-column injury. The anterior longitudinal ligament, posterior longitudinal ligament, disc annulus, facet capsules, and interspinous ligaments are all disrupted. These patients commonly present with significant neurologic deficit. A more extreme form of this type of injury is cervical spondyloptosis, which is pictured preoperatively in **Fig. 5–3** and postoperatively in **Fig. 5–4**. These patients are quadriplegic, and by definition the upper segment is 100% subluxed in relation to the lower segment.

Complete spine precautions must be practiced, and hypoxia and hypotension should be avoided. The rest of the spine should also be evaluated for concomitant injury, especially in these cases. Multisystem trauma can result from the degree of force responsible for this type of injury and must be carefully sought out. Methylprednisolone spinal cord injury protocol should be started if the patient presented within 8 hours of injury.

After an emergency magnetic resonance imaging (MRI), if there is no acute disc compressing the cord, closed reduction can be attempted through careful coaxial traction. Because the patient will require operative fixation, open reduction can be achieved surgically, but this takes away the advantage of an immediate postreduction examination. If a compressive disc herniation is identified on MRI, emergency surgery for decompression and stabilization is done. This may require an anterior discectomy, posterior fusion, and then anterior fusion. Alternatively, it may require only an anterior discectomy and fusion, followed by a posterior fusion if reduction has been achieved. Drilling the facets posteriorly and realigning the spine after the anterior discectomy help in posterior reduction. All maneuvering of these patients needs to be done with the utmost care, as all manipulation carries the risk of greater damage to the cord. If reduction is done while the patient is under anesthesia, it is prudent to have neurophysiologic monitoring.

SUGGESTED READING

Selden NR, Quint DJ, Patel N, d'Arcy HS, Papadopoulos SM. Emergency magnetic resonance imaging of cervical spinal cord injuries: clinical correlation and prognosis. Neurosurgery 1999;44:785–792

6

Cervical Kyphosis

■ Presentation

A 46-year-old man injured his neck as a child and was quadriplegic for 6 months, but recovered. Over recent years he complained of neck pain and progressive kyphosis. He had myelopathic signs on examination.

■ Radiologic Findings

T2-weighted magnetic resonance imaging (MRI) of the cervical spine (**Fig. 6–1**) displays a compressed, retropulsed C7 vertebral body, with cervical kyphosis and cord compression.

■ Diagnosis

Cervical deformity

■ Treatment

A two-level cervical corpectomy with insertion of titanium cage was accomplished under axial traction.

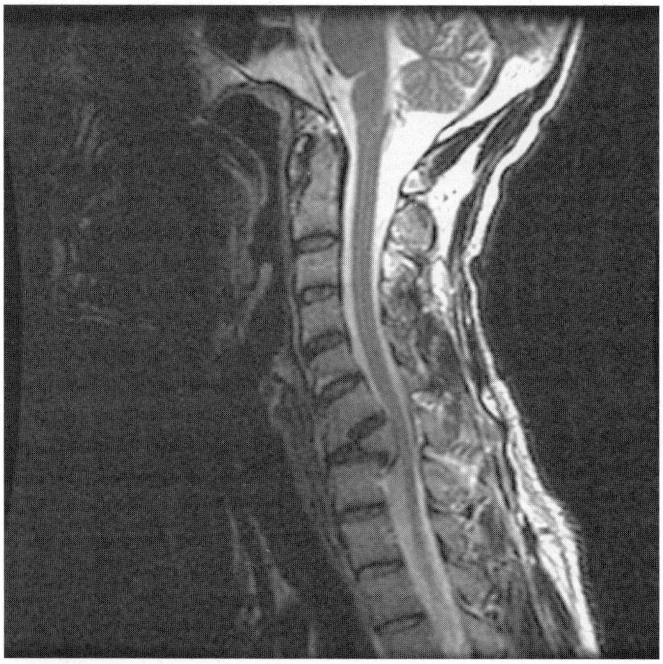

FIGURE 6–1 Sagittal T2-weighted MRI shows a severely compressed C7 vertebral body impinging on the cord with cervical kyphosis.

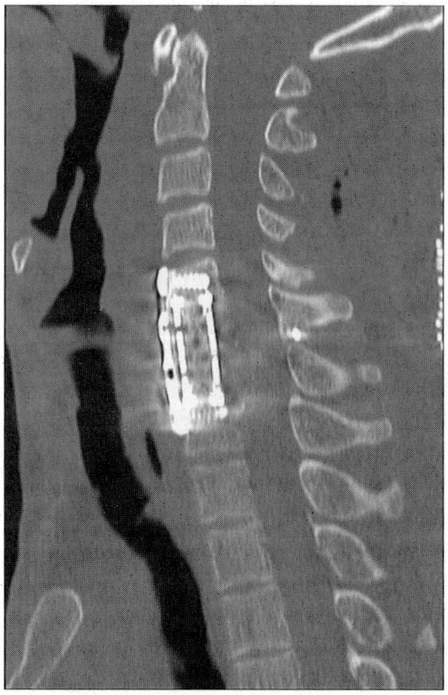

FIGURE 6–2 Postoperative CT scan demonstrates a two-level corpectomy with allograft and instrumentation.

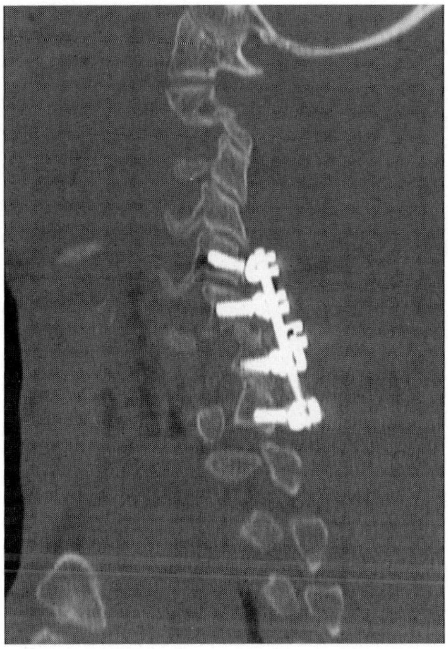

FIGURE 6–3 Postoperative CT scan displays a posterior cervical fusion with lateral mass plates spanning C5 to T1.

This was followed by posterior fusion and instrumentation (360-degree fusion). The postoperative construct can be seen on sagittal reconstructed cervical computed tomography (CT) in **Figs. 6–2** and **6–3**.

■ Discussion

Many factors are considered in determining when to use an anterior cervical approach. One must study the cervical contour and alignment, noting the presence or absence of severe kyphosis. The nature of the compression, whether it is ventrally located, and its components—central or paracentral disc herniation, calcified disc or hard bony osteophytes, short segmental ossification of the posterior longitudinal ligament, or vertebral body pathology (fracture, tumor)—would direct one toward an anterior approach. The number of segments fused is another factor. A one- or two-level corpectomy can be managed anteriorly alone with good fusion rate. On the other hand, a three-or-more-level corpectomy is associated with a significantly higher rate of pseudarthrosis and hardware failure unless a posterior tension band is added. Other considerations are the patient's overall and cardiac health, activity level, bone quality, and nicotine use. The surgeon should be experienced in the general approach as well.

This patient likely developed a teardrop fracture with loss of lordosis as a child that healed with prolonged bed rest. As he aged and degenerative changes occurred, his deformity was exaggerated to the point of neurologic compromise. In the case of such significant kyphosis and compression, anterior decompression and fusion would not alone correct his imbalance. In addition, the nonfusion rate increases with multilevel corpectomies. A posterior tension band is needed for correction, strength, and to enhance arthrodesis.

SUGGESTED READING

Liew SM, Simmons Ed Jr. Cervical deformity: rationale for selecting the appropriate fusion technique (anterior, posterior, and 360 degree). Orthop Clin North Am 1998;29:779–786

7

Spinal Trauma

Presentation

A 17-year-old boy was in a motor vehicle accident and became paraplegic. He had a cervical fusion for stabilization and then extensive rehabilitation. During his rehabilitation course, a urinary tract infection seeded his epidural space, causing a discitis and osteomyelitis (**Fig. 7–1**). This was treated with prolonged intravenous antibiotics. A couple years after his accident, he began experiencing worsening hand weakness, paresthesias, and hyperhidrosis.

Radiologic Findings

Magnetic resonance imaging (MRI) of the cervical spine shows an intramedullary fluid-filled cavity at C7–T1 (**Fig. 7–2**). There is also some metallic artifact seen around the posterior elements from the patient's previous fusion.

Diagnosis

Posttraumatic syrinx

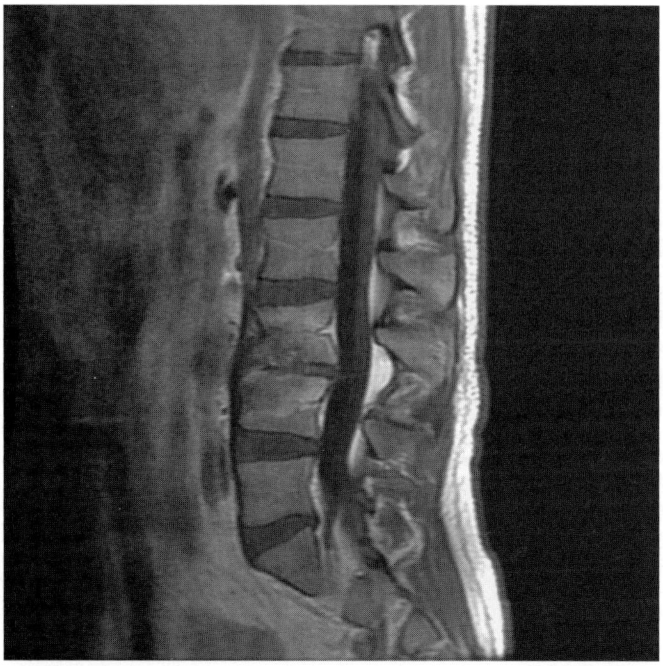

FIGURE 7–1 Lumbar MRI with L3–L4 osteomyelitis and discitis.

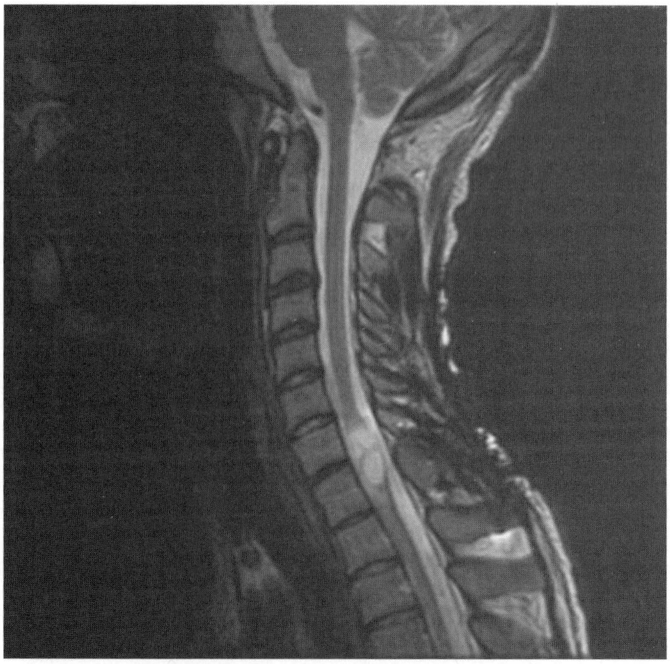

FIGURE 7–2 Posttraumatic cervicothoracic syrinx.

■ Treatment

The patient received a syringosubarachnoid shunt with adhesiolysis.

■ Discussion

The occurrence of posttraumatic syringomyelia is ~5%. This may occur a few months following injury, but usually occurs years later. The etiology is believed to be the coalescence of multiple microcysts at the site of the initial cord contusion, combined with the tethering effect of surrounding adhesions.

Clinically the diagnosis is suspected by the development of new, intense, dysesthetic pains in the most rostral area of dysfunction. The pain is exacerbated by Valsalva maneuvers such as coughing or sneezing. On examination, findings of delayed neurologic deficit, increased weakness in lower extremities, spasticity, an ascending sensory level, loss of previously functioning muscle groups, and deterioration of bowel and bladder dysfunction are typical. Hyperhidrosis is also frequently reported.

Additionally complicating this patient's picture is his history of discitis. It is possible that he may have infected another area of the spine, causing his current neurologic deterioration. A full-spine MRI ruled out this diagnosis, but revealed the aforementioned syrinx.

Patients with these symptoms need a spinal MRI or computed tomography (CT) myelogram if the metallic artifact is too great. Percutaneous aspiration of the syrinx is challenging and only a temporizing measure. Surgical intervention to lyse adhesions and divert the syrinx fluid into a normal area of subarachnoid space a few segments caudal to the pathology is more successful. However stabilizing it is hoped the surgery will be, the natural history of a posttraumatic syrinx is one of continuous deterioration over time.

SUGGESTED READING

Kramer KM, Levine AM. Posttraumatic syringomyelia: a review of 21 cases. Clin Orthop Relat Res 1997;334:190–199

8

Ankylosing Spondylitis

■ Presentation

A 72-year-old man with ankylosing spondylitis slipped on the ice and fell. He went to the emergency department 3 days later with neck pain.

■ Radiologic Findings

A chance-like fracture is seen on cervical x-ray at C5, splitting the spine into two autofused segments above and below the injury, rendering the patient grossly unstable (**Fig. 8–1**). In addition, **Fig. 8–2** demonstrates the long arm autofusion typical of ankylosing spondylitis, extending throughout his thoracic spine on x-ray. This has been referred to as a "bamboo spine" (**Fig. 8–2**).

■ Diagnosis

Unstable cervical fracture with ankylosing spondylitis

■ Treatment

Cervical realignment and fusion (**Fig. 8–3**)

■ Discussion

Ankylosing spondylitis is a human leukocyte antigen (HLA)–B27-seronegative arthritis with the main pathology occurring at bony attachment of ligaments, tendons, and capsules. These sites undergo inflammation and then calcification and ossification. Sacroiliac joints, the greater trochanter, patella, and spine are classic areas of involvement and their ossification can be seen on x-ray. Gradual loss of spine and sacroiliac mobility, arthritis, uveitis, aortic intimal changes, and renal and pulmonary issues are the main highlights of this disease. The inflammatory process is slowly progressive and

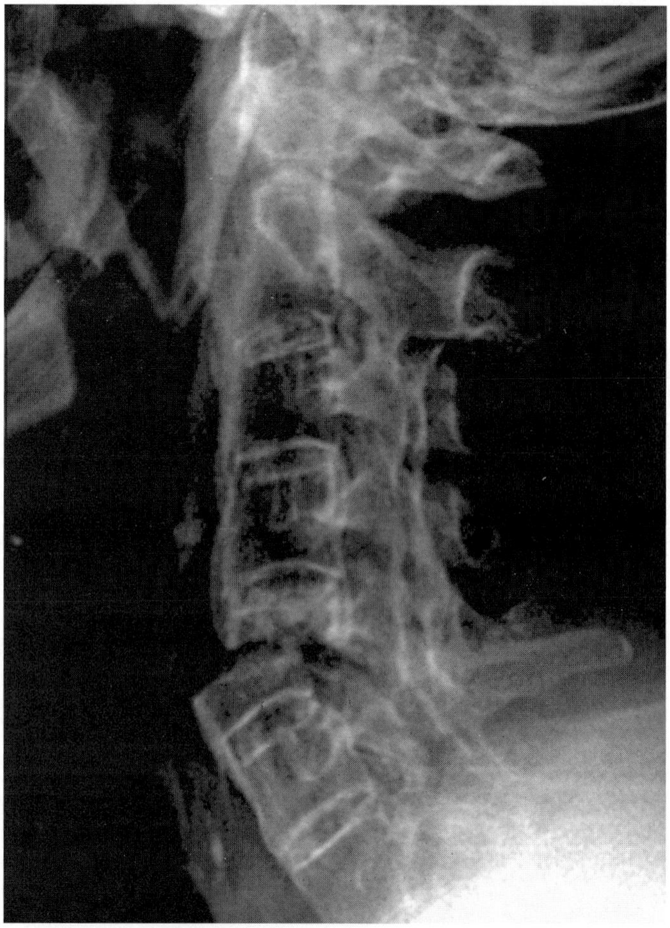

FIGURE 8–1 Unstable three-column C5 fracture through the C5 body and into the posterior elements with separate long moment arms above and below.

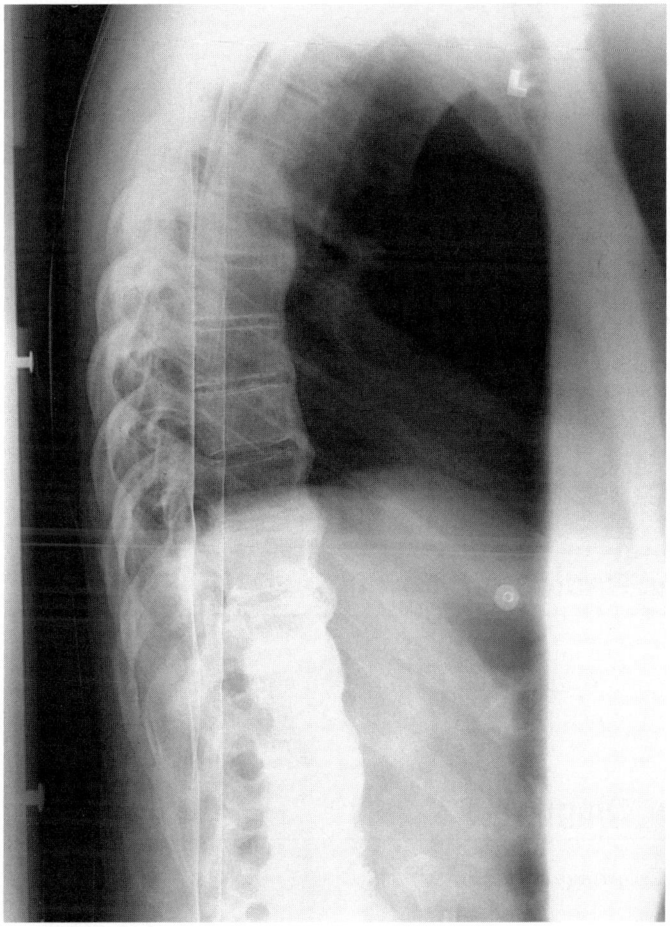

FIGURE 8–2 Thoracic x-ray with osteophytic bridging typical of ankylosing spondylitis.

anti-inflammatory medication and physiotherapy are the mainstays of treatment.

Ankylosing spondylitis affects males more than females and is usually discovered in adolescence or young adulthood. As the disease evolves, patients get increasingly kyphosed, leading to more falls, and they eventually lose the ability to guard against further falls. This perpetuates a dangerous cycle. Minimal trauma causes significant spinal fractures as the bone is brittle

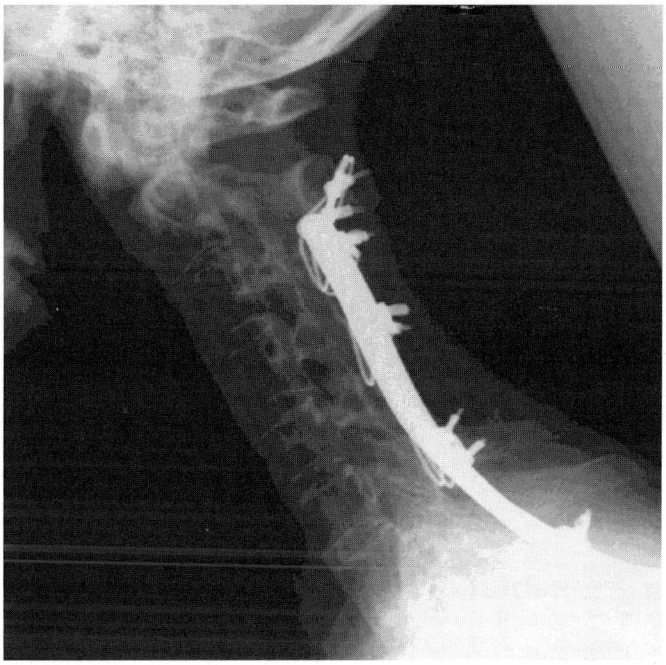

FIGURE 8–3 Postoperative construct as seen on cervical x-ray.

and the spine has autofused. Spine fractures are typically three-column injuries resulting in listhesis and often associated with an epidural hematoma.

Dorsal corrective fusion surgery is the procedure of choice, but the bone quality in these patients is poor, and a 360-degree fusion may be needed. Also, complicating surgery is difficulty in positioning, secondary to preexisting deformity and the fragility of the spine. Intraoperatively, rampant ossification affects the appearance of classic spinal landmarks. Because of a patient's fall and pseudarthrosis risk, postoperative orthosis is necessary.

SUGGESTED READING

Koh WH, Garrett SL, Calin A. Cervical spine surgery in ankylosing spondylitis: is the outcome good? Clin Rheumatol 1997; 16:466–470

9

Esophageal Injury

■ Presentation

A 70-year-old man fell down a flight of stairs, sustaining an incomplete cervical spinal cord injury. He had a three-column C4 fracture and radiologic findings of ankylosing spondylitis. He was taken to the operating room and reduced and fused anteriorly and posteriorly. Postoperatively, a neck abscess was discovered during a febrile workup. This was surgically explored, and a communication between the esophagus and surrounding neck tissue was found.

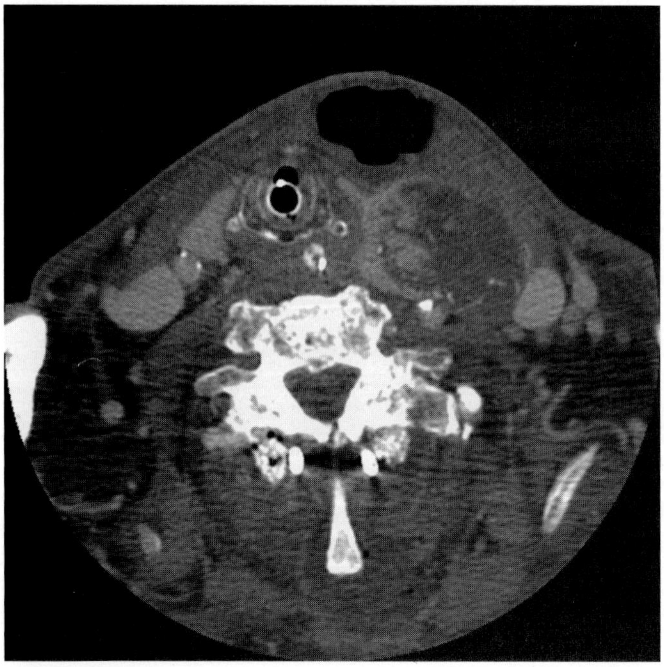

FIGURE 9–1 CT soft tissue of the neck shows a left-sided abscess.

■ Radiologic Findings

A left anterior neck abscess is seen on this contrast-enhanced soft tissue computed tomography (CT) scan of the neck (**Fig. 9–1**).

■ Diagnosis

Esophageal fistula

■ Treatment

Surgical debridement and external drainage were done in conjunction with the ear, nose, and throat surgeons.

■ Discussion

While more commonly seen in penetrating neck trauma, an esophageal injury may also have been reported following traumatic injury to cervical spine. The cause can be multifactorial; an esophageal laceration by a sharp bony edge at the fracture site is typically the offending pathology. It is also possible to cause such injury iatrogenically.

These injuries are difficult to diagnose preoperatively because the patient may be intubated and unable to communicate, and more acute symptomatic injuries (spinal cord injury) are the initial focus.

Often, esophageal injury is diagnosed later, during the search for an infectious source. Primary repair is difficult; the exact site of injury can be distorted due to tissue swelling, infection, and its small size. Treatment consists of primary or flap repair if possible, debridement, drainage, and a long course of intravenous antibiotics covering aerobes and anaerobes. It is not necessary to remove the hardware, as the risks of destabilization outweigh the benefits. In this case, the hardware was left in, and the patient ultimately recovered from his abscess.

SUGGESTED READING

Gaudinez RF, English GM, Gebhard JS, Brugman JL, Donaldson DH, Brown CW. Esophageal perforations after anterior cervical surgery. J Spinal Disord 2000;13:77–84

10

Traumatic Thoracic Fracture

■ Presentation

An 18-year-old man had a rollover motor vehicle accident and presented with a complete T4 spinal cord injury. The instability of his spine would have made nursing care and rehabilitation activity difficult, so he underwent surgical stabilization.

■ Radiologic Findings

Sagittal magnetic resonance imaging (MRI) of his thoracic spine is most significant for a T2–T3 fracture dislocation that affected all three columns (**Fig. 10–1**).

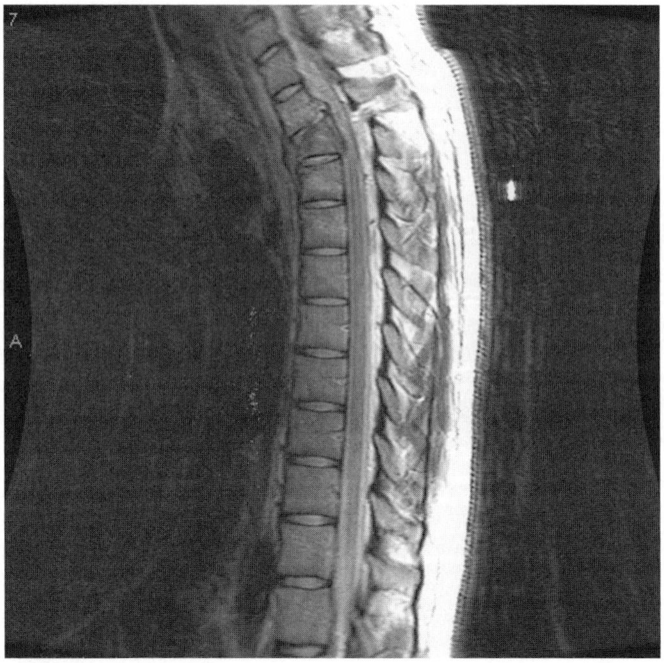

FIGURE 10–1 MRI of the thoracic spine reveals a T2–T3 fracture dislocation.

■ Diagnosis

Unstable thoracic fracture

■ Treatment

A multilevel cervicothoracic reconstruction was completed, as seen in **Fig. 10–2**. Note that the patient also

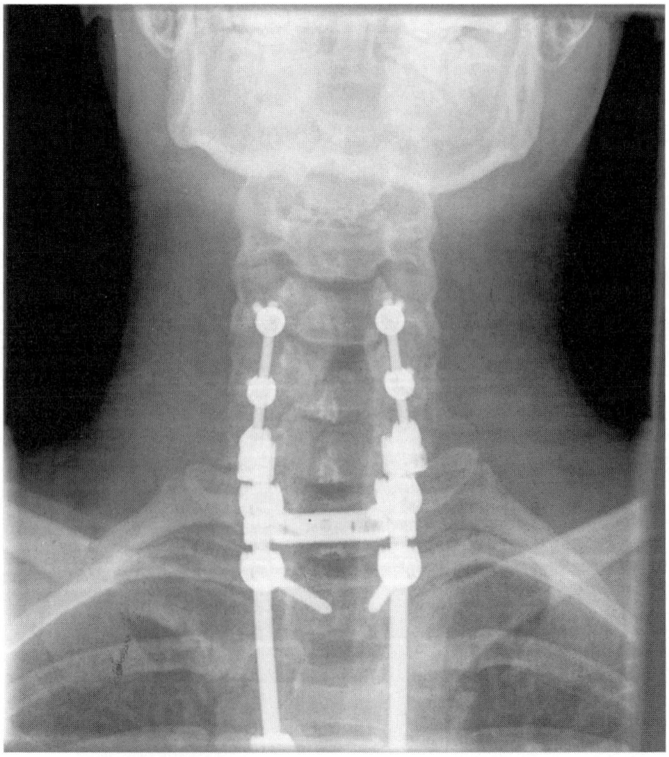

FIGURE 10–2 Postoperative construct is seen on anteroposterior (AP) x-ray.

had a C5–C6 facet fracture that necessitated cephalad extension of the fusion.

■ Discussion

The three-column model of Denis provides for an anterior column (the anterior longitudinal ligament and annulus, and anterior portion of the vertebral body), the middle column (posterior longitudinal ligament and annulus, and posterior portion of the vertebral body), and the posterior column (all the rest of the posterior structures). Any injury that affects two or more columns renders the spine unstable, often needs fixation, and may involve neurologic compromise.

Multiple classification themes are described to categorize thoracolumbar fractures. The most reliable and widely used is the Comprehensive Classification of Thoracic and Lumbar Spine Injuries. It is based in the mechanism of injury and the vectors of force—distraction, compression, and multidirectional with translation (**Table 10–1**).

There are four more commonly seen thoracic and lumbar fractures: (1) a compression fracture involves the anterior column and occurs from an axial flexion force; (2) a burst fracture results from an axial load that damages the anterior and middle columns; (3) a chance fracture, frequently referred to as a "seat-belt fracture," is a flexion distraction injury that occurs when the upper body is thrown forward and the pelvis remains stable; three-column damage ensues; and (4) a fracture dislocation is another three-column injury that involves one vertebra becoming displaced from alignment, usually through rotational forces.

TABLE 10–1 Thoracolumbar Injury Classification Based on the Association for the Study of Internal Fixation (AO/ASIF) Criteria

Type	*Group*
Compression	Impaction fracture Split fracture Burst fracture
Distraction	Posterior soft tissue disruption Posterior arch fracture Anteriorly through disk
Multidirectional with translation	Anteroposterior Lateral Rotational

SUGGESTED READINGS

Croce MA, Bee TK, Pritchard E, Miler PR, Fabian TC. Does optimal timing for spinal fracture fixation exist? Ann Surg 2001;233:851–858

Magerl F, Aebi M, Gertzbein SD, Harms J, Nazarian S. A comprehensive classification of thoracic and lumbar injuries. Eur Spine J 1994;3:184–201

11

Lumbar Fracture

■ Presentation

A 52-year-old man fell the height of one story a year ago. He has had chronic low back pain since then. His neurologic examination is normal.

■ Radiologic Findings

An L2 wedge fracture is seen on computed tomography (CT) reconstruction, with associated kyphosis (**Fig. 11–1**).

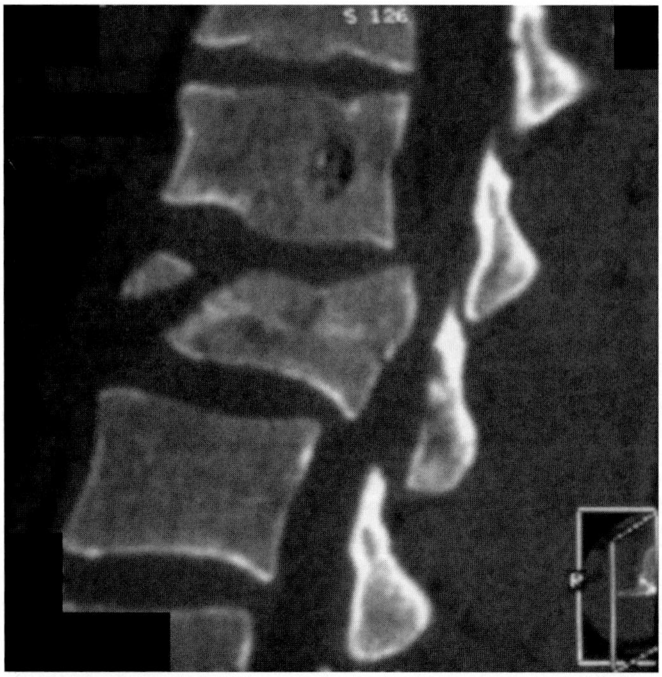

FIGURE 11–1 CT reconstruction of the lumbar spine with an L2 wedge compression fracture and kyphosis is seen.

■ Diagnosis

Wedge compression fracture

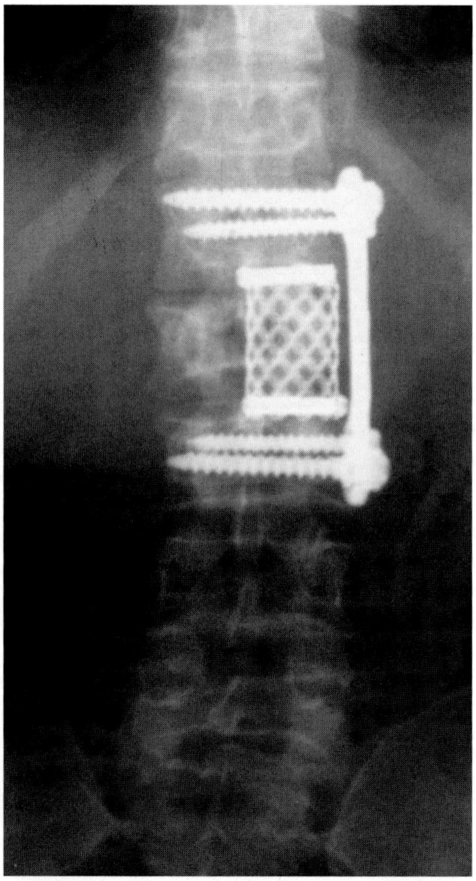

FIGURE 11–2 Postoperative anteroposterior (AP) x-ray reveals the fusion construct.

■ Treatment

A left-sided retroperitoneal approach was used for an L2 corpectomy with cage and plate stabilization (**Fig. 11–2**).

■ Discussion

Flexion compression fractures (wedge fracture) cause failure of the anterior column. They are the most common type of thoracic and lumbar fracture. Denis divides these fractures into four subtypes. They are listed by decreasing frequency: fracture of the superior end plate, fracture of both end plates with separation of the anterior body, fracture of the anterior surface with end plates intact, and fracture of the inferior end plate. These are usually stable fractures. Patients should receive analgesics and early mobilization.

Surgery is indicated if patients develop progressive kyphosis. Patients at risk to develop progressive kyphosis from a compression wedge fracture have a 50% loss of vertebral body height, over 30 degrees of angulation, or failure of the posterior column. Posterior column failure can also be iatrogenic in etiology, stemming from a previous laminectomy.

An anterior approach (retroperitoneal) can be used in thoracolumbar junction fractures to better decompress a stenosed canal, support the anterior column, and enhance fusion rate without incorporating a long-arm segment. Bicortical screw purchase is necessary to stabilize this junctional segment. The disadvantages are that the procedure carries a relatively high morbidity and is technically demanding.

SUGGESTED READING

Denis F. The three column spine and its significance in the classification of acute thoracolumbar spinal injuries. Spine 1983;8:817–831

12

Burst Fracture

■ Presentation

A 50-year-old woman fell 15 feet and developed lower thoracic pain that did not improve. The pain was axial, without radiation. She did not have any deficit on examination.

■ Radiologic Findings

A T11 burst fracture is featured on reconstructed (**Fig. 12–1**) and axial thoracolumbar computed tomography (CT) scan (**Fig. 12–2**).

■ Diagnosis

Thoracic burst fracture

■ Treatment

A thoracic fusion was completed.

■ Discussion

Burst fractures constitute 20% of major spine injuries. They are a two-column injury. A burst fracture is

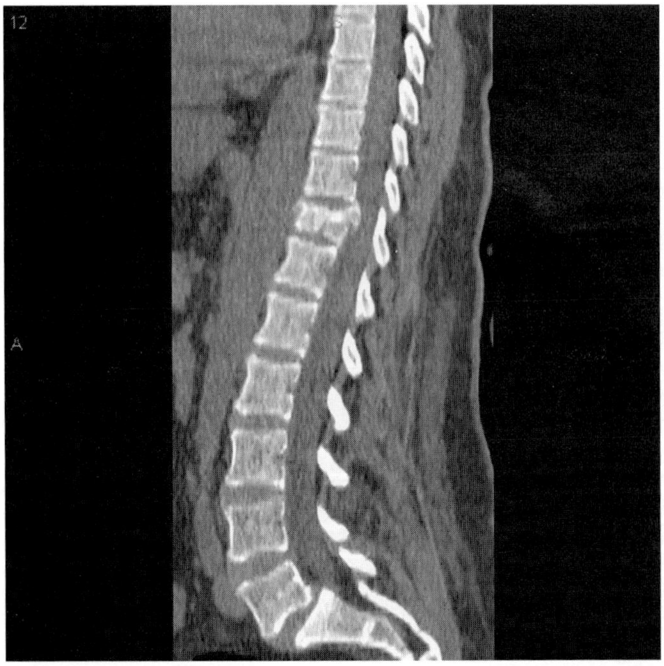

FIGURE 12–1 Sagittal reconstruction demonstrates a T11 fracture with 50% loss of height and 50% canal compromise.

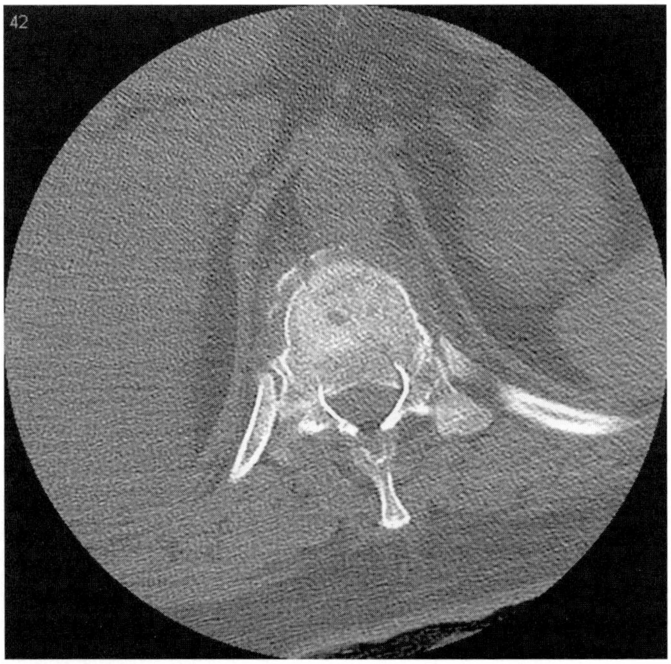

FIGURE 12–2 Axial CT slice through T11.

differentiated from a compression fracture by the presence of posterior vertebral body line failure, retropulsion, and widening of the interpedicular distance, indicating failure of the anterior and middle columns. This is usually associated with incomplete neurologic deficit.

When considering the treatment for a burst fracture, the issues are the role of surgery, decompression or stabilization, or both. If the fracture has more than 50% loss of vertebral body height, 50% canal compromise, or more than 30 degrees of angulation, fusion is recommended. On the other hand, some studies have demonstrated bone healing without significant deformity if no intervention is done on these patients.

Surgical decompression is required if there is evidence of continued radiologic compression in patients with an incomplete neurologic deficit. Decompression is not indicated in patients with complete spinal cord injury, regardless of the status of the canal; however, it is frequently performed when a patient is undergoing a stabilization procedure.

SUGGESTED READING

Wood K, Butterman G, Mehbod A, Garvey T, Jhanjee R, Sechriest V. Operative compared with nonoperative treatment of a thoracolumbar burst fracture without neurological deficit. A prospective, randomized study. J Bone Joint Surg Am 2003;85-A:773–781

13

Traumatic Lumbar Fracture

■ Presentation

An 18-year-old woman was hit by a car and sustained multisystemic injury. On presentation she was paraplegic and had complete spinal cord injury in the lower extremities. She had a prolonged intensive care unit course and was finally stable enough for surgery.

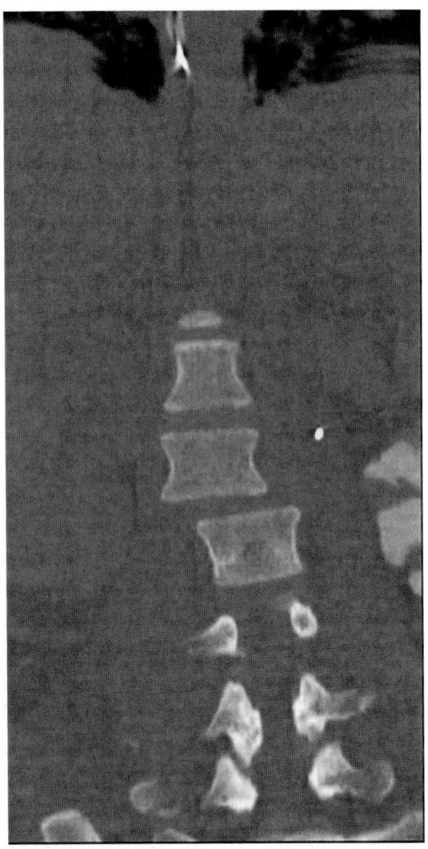

FIGURE 13–1 CT AP reconstruction of the thoracolumbar junction shows an L1–L2 fracture dislocation.

■ Radiologic Findings

Anteroposterior (AP) reconstruction of the thoracolumbar junction shows an L1–L2 fracture dislocation. An axial slice through the area demonstrates the rotational translation of L1 on L2 (**Figs. 13–1** and **13–2**).

■ Diagnosis

Fracture dislocation of the lumbar spine

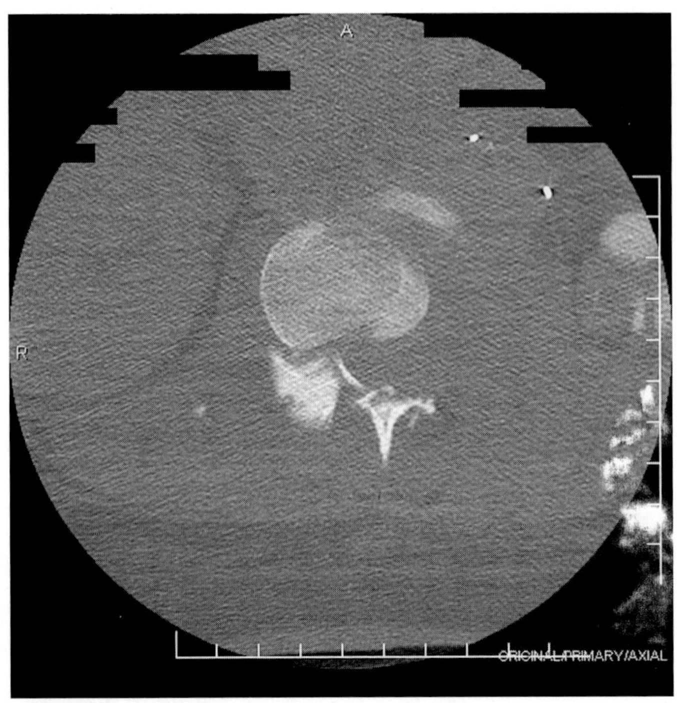

FIGURE 13–2 An axial CT slice through the area demonstrates the rotational translation of L1 on L2.

TABLE 13–1 The Surgical Approaches to the Spine

Approach/Level	*Ventral*	*Ventrolateral*	*Dorsolateral*	*Dorsal*
C6–T3	Cervicothoracic	—	Lat. parascapular extrapleural	Transpedicular Translaminar
T3–T10	Transthoracic	Retropleural	Lat. extracavitary	Transpedicular Translaminar
T10–L5	Thoracoabdominal	Retroperitoneal	Costotransversectomy	Transpedicular Translaminar

■ Treatment

Decompression, reduction, and thoracolumbar pedicle screw fixation were undertaken through a posterior approach.

■ Discussion

Fracture dislocations of the spine are the result of severe forces that disrupt all three columns by combining rotation, tension, compression, and shear. Flexion rotation fractures often occur through the disc space. These are associated with abdominal injury and neurologic damage. Treatment focuses on realignment of the spinal column, posterior stabilization, and early mobilization.

The surgical approach of a thoracolumbar fracture depends on location, mechanism of injury, neurologic status, and overall clinical status. **Table 13–1** summarizes the approaches.

SUGGESTED READING

Chaloupka R. Complete rotational burst fracture of the third lumbar vertebra managed by posterior surgery. A case report. Spine 1999;24:302–305

14

Multiple Burst Fractures

■ Presentation

A 25-year-old man was skydiving and missed his optimal landing site, injuring himself. He complained of low back pain, but had no neurologic deficit.

■ Radiologic Findings

Figs. 14–1 and **14–2** demonstrate L1 and L4 burst fractures on sagittal lumbar computed tomography (CT) reconstruction.

■ Diagnosis

Multiple lumbar burst fractures

■ Treatment

The patient underwent long-arm fusion. The postoperative construct can be seen on anteroposterior (AP) lumbar x-ray in **Fig. 14–3**.

■ Discussion

There is a spectrum of opinion in the spine literature regarding optimum treatment for vertebral body compression fractures. This ranges from conservative therapy to anterior, posterior, or combined approaches. Generally, surgery is accepted as the mainstay for patients with an incomplete deficit or radiographic signs suggesting an incompetent posterior column—over 25 degrees of kyphosis, fanning of the spinous processes, or facet separation.

An anterior approach affords a better chance of decompression with a more sound structural reconstruction. This technique would be ideal for a comminuted vertebral body fracture ranging from T11 to L3. On the

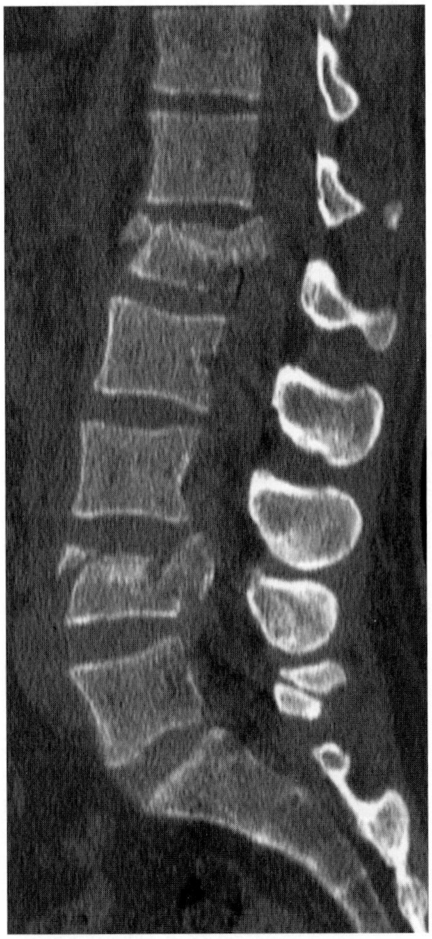

FIGURE 14–1 Sagittal CT reconstruction demonstrating L1 and L4 burst fractures.

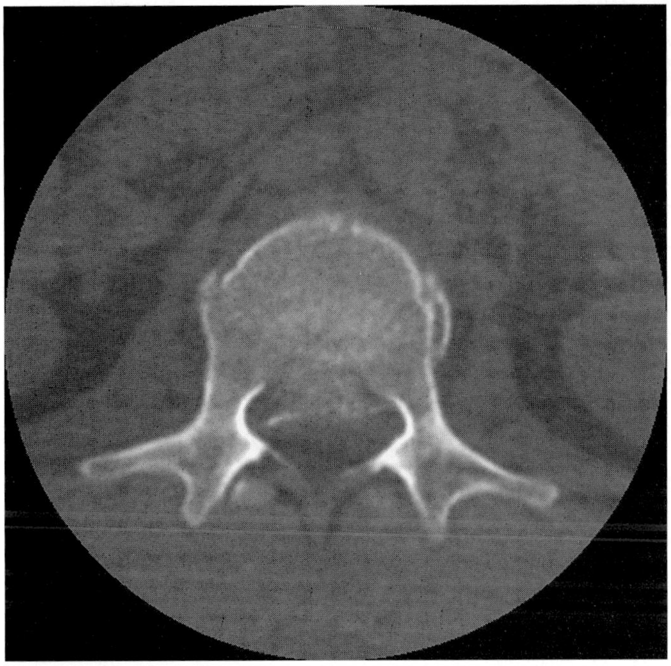

FIGURE 14–2 Axial CT through the L4 burst fracture.

other hand, the morbidity of this approach, especially in the acute trauma setting, can be quite significant. The anterior approach is contraindicated in osteoporotic patients, abdominal trauma, a failed posterior tension band, and nerve root entrapment. The posterior approach is faster, more familiar to many spine surgeons, less morbid, and often adequate. It is more appropriate for lower lumbar injuries, as the psoas muscle and major vessels become major ventral surgical obstacles in this region. Simple bracing without surgery escalates morbidities such as deep venous thrombosis and pneumonia, prevents early mobilization, and increases time off from work.

The challenge of this case is the combination of a thoracolumbar fracture and lower lumbar fracture. This necessitates a longer fusion arm. Incorporation of the S1 segment is essential here to avoid the disadvantages of "floating fusion." Because the patient was neurologically intact a corpectomy was not indicated, we felt a posterior procedure would suffice.

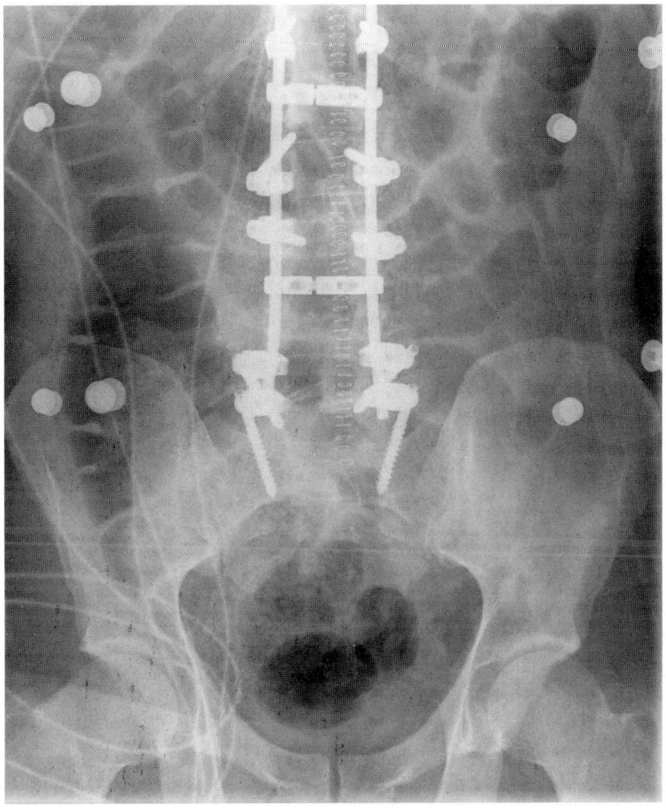

FIGURE 14–3 Postoperative construct.

SUGGESTED READING

Finkenberg J, Banta C, Cross GL 3rd, et al. Evaluation and analysis of patient outcomes with an intrasegmental fixation system in lumbar spinal fusion. Spine J 2001;1:102–108

15

Sacral Fracture

RAHUL VAIDYA AND MARILYN GATES

■ Presentation

A 64-year-old man fell and complained of sacral pain. He was neurologically intact, including bowel and bladder function.

■ Radiologic Findings

Fig. 15–1, a sagittal computed tomography (CT) reconstruction of the lumbosacral spine, is notable for a traumatic listhesis of S1 on S2.

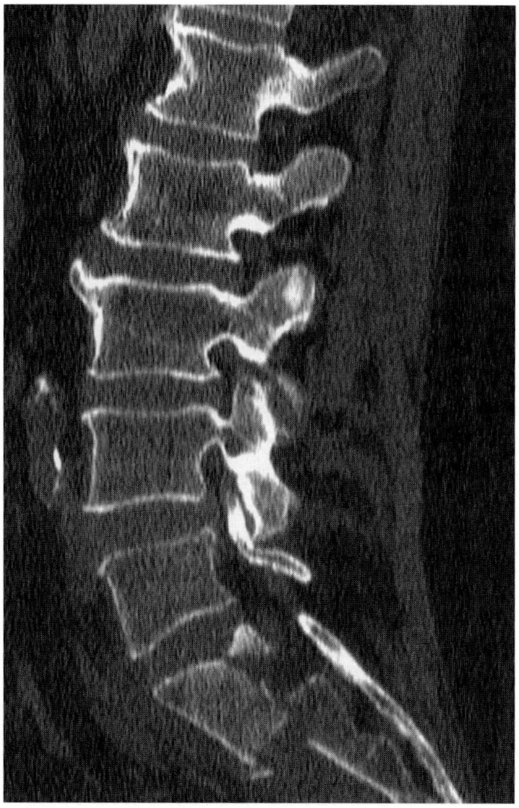

FIGURE 15–1 A comminuted, displaced fracture incorporating S1 and S2 is seen on CT.

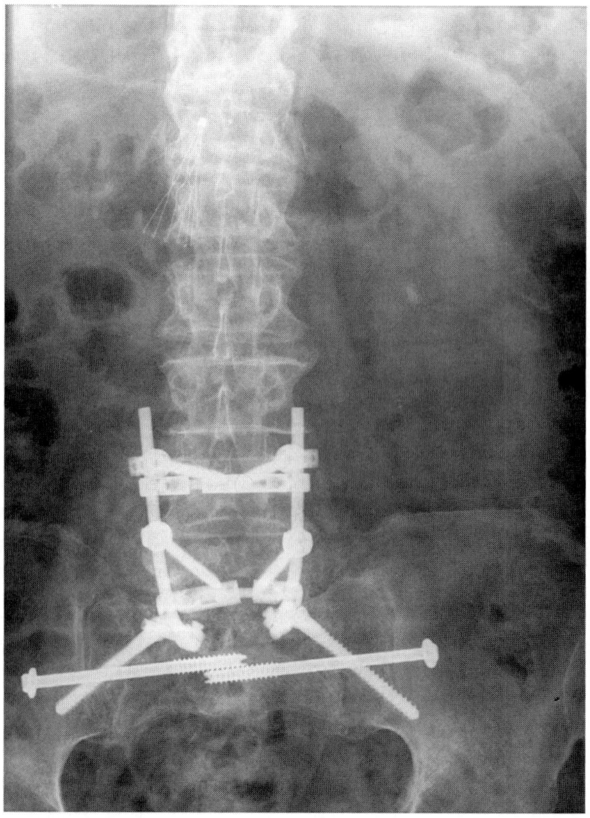

FIGURE 15–2 Postoperative x-ray showing lumbopelvic fixation.

■ Diagnosis

Traumatic sacral fracture, zone III

■ Treatment

A lumbosacral fixation was performed (**Fig. 15–2**).

■ Discussion

Sacral fractures are classified according to zone. Zone I is across the ala and can cause L5 impingement. Zone II is through the neural foramina and may result in a unilateral sacral anesthesia. Zone III is through the body of the sacrum and is most likely to injure the cauda.

A neurologic examination should be done to assess for neural compromise, including bowel and bladder function. The fracture stability must be determined by looking at the arcuate lines on pelvic x-ray and CT scan to better delineate the fracture extent. Zone I fractures may heal with traction and rest. Zone II injuries require operative debridement of the fracture fragments prior to posterior reduction and fixation. Zone III fractures also need decompression and fusion.

Lumbopelvic fusion, using any of the available systems for sacroiliac fixation, is appropriate. In this case, the lumbar spine was fixated with pedicle screws, which were joined through a rod to iliac wing screws. The patient then had bilateral sacroiliac screws for additional sacral fixation. He was non–weight-bearing for 3 months.

SUGGESTED READING

Taguchi T, Kawai S, Kaneko K, Yugue D. Operative management of displaced fractures of the sacrum. J Orthop Sci 1999;4:347–352

16

Atlanto-occipital Dislocation

ERIC SPICKLER

▪ Presentation

A 20-year-old woman was hit by a car and presented comatose, in cardiac arrest.

▪ Radiologic Findings

Sagittal reconstructed computed tomography (CT) of the cervical spine is notable for craniocervical dislocation (**Fig. 16–1**).

▪ Diagnosis

Atlanto-occipital dislocation

▪ Treatment

Although the patient's vital signs were revived, she was declared brain dead.

▪ Discussion

Atlanto-occipital dislocation is a common site of fatal injury in children sustaining significant upper cervical trauma. The fatality results from a hyperextension-distraction injury of the craniocervical junction leading to shearing of the cervicomedullary junction and respiratory arrest. While the mechanism is typically traumatic, it may be encountered in atraumatic cases such as Down syndrome or rheumatoid arthritis. The tectorial ligaments, which hold the condyles to the atlas, are torn.

Atlanto-occipital dislocation is a radiographic diagnosis. Several measurements are described to establish the diagnosis. However, the condition is often grossly evident based on radiographs, the patient's poor clinical condition, and the mechanism of injury. The Powers ratio takes the distance from the basion to the midvertical portion of the posterior laminar line of the atlas (BC), over the distance from the opisthion to the midvertical

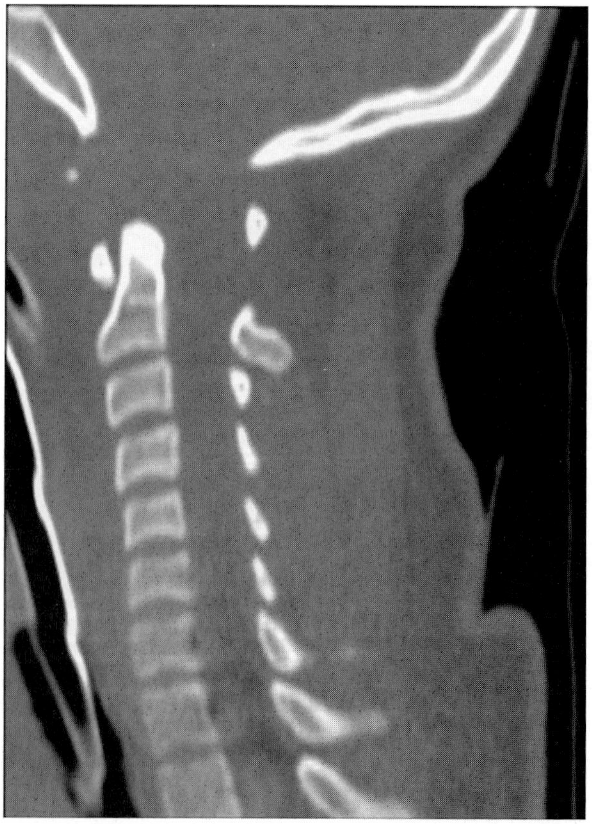

FIGURE 16–1 Sagittal CT reconstruction of the cervical spine shows a Powers ratio above 1, verifying grossly notable atlanto-occipital dislocation.

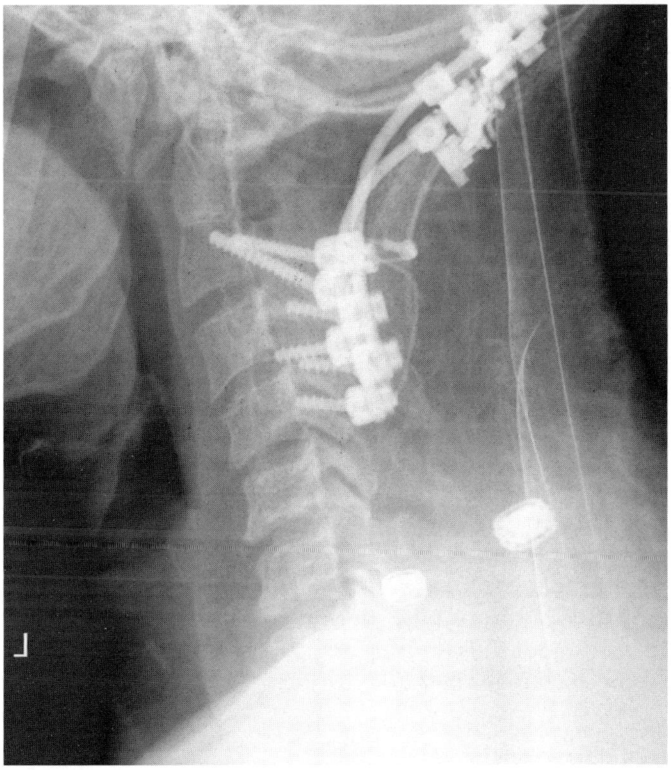

FIGURE 17–3 Lateral C-spine x-ray displays an occipitocervical fusion with rib autograft.

■ Discussion

Platybasia refers to the flattening of the skull base and can occur congenitally, with Chiari malformation, Paget's disease, and rheumatoid arthritis. Platybasia is demonstrated when a line can be drawn from the nasion to the tuberculum sella and then to the anterior foramen magnum, and the angle is greater than 143 degrees.

This often occurs in conjunction with cranial settling, otherwise known as basilar invagination. This can be measured by a series of lines. McGregor's line is drawn from the hard palate to the posterior occiput curve. If the tip of the dens is more than 4.5 mm above this line, there is cranial settling. Ranwat's line is drawn from the center of the C2 pedicle to a line connecting the anterior and posterior C1 arches. If this distance is less than 13 mm, there is basilar invagination.

There are many different posterior instrumentation systems designed for occipitocervical fusion, as well as a sundry array of graft substitutes. This patient received a screw and rod system bent to accommodate the sharp angle of the occipitocervical junction. A rib autograft was also fashioned to accommodate the natural curve of the area. On follow-up the patient had returned to functioning and had a solid fusion.

SUGGESTED READING

Riew KD, Hilibrand AS, Palumbo MA, Sethi N, Bohlman HH. Diagnosing basilar invagination in the rheumatoid patient. The reliability of radiographic criteria. J Bone Joint Surg Am 2001; 83-A:194–200

18

Rheumatoid Arthritis

■ Presentation

A 74-year-old woman was admitted to the hospital after a simple fall. Magnetic resonance imaging (MRI) revealed posterior upper cervical cord compression secondary to C1–C2 anterior subluxation. She did not have any neurologic deficit.

■ Radiologic Findings

On MRI there is marked compression of the cervical spinal cord at the craniocervical junction with basilar invagination and a C1 fracture (**Fig. 18–1**). Computed tomography (CT) and x-ray further delineate the anterior dislocation of C1. There is basilar invagination and narrowing of the cervical canal (**Figs. 18–2** and **18–3**). All of these changes looked chronic.

■ Diagnosis

Chronic cervical pathology, relating to rheumatoid arthritis

■ Treatment

The patient was fitted with a cervical collar.

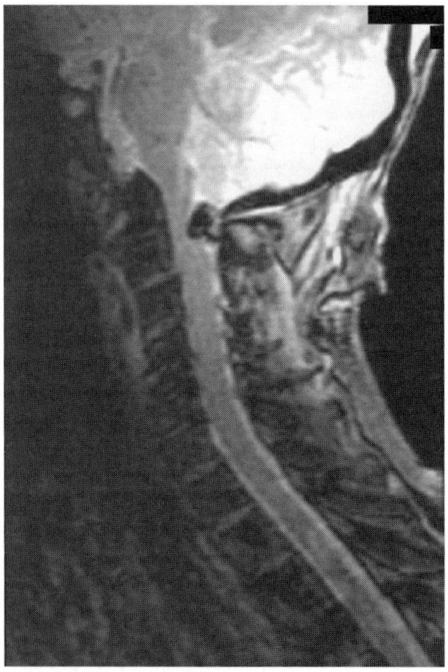

FIGURE 18–1 MRI with basilar invagination.

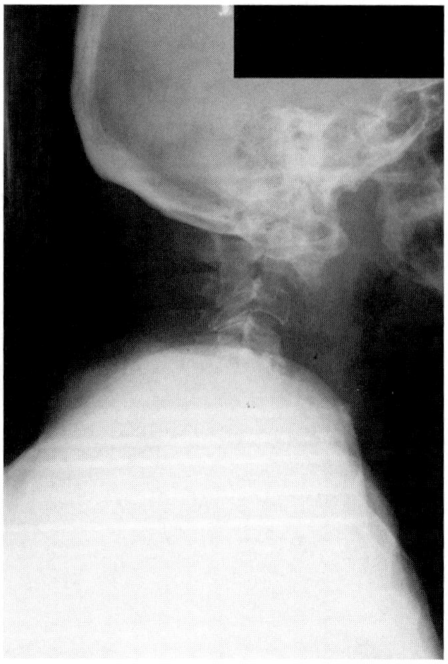

FIGURE 18–2 Lateral C-spine x-ray is noteworthy for basilar invagination.

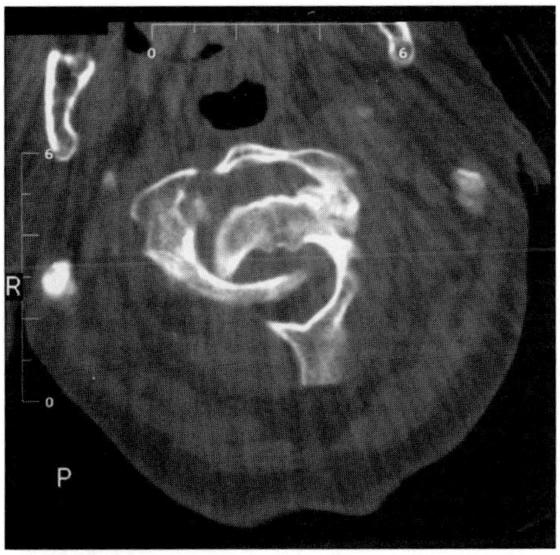

FIGURE 18–3 Axial cut CT the C-spine shows the atlantoaxial dislocation.

■ Discussion

Anterior atlantoaxial subluxation and basilar impression are common in rheumatoid arthritis. As synovial proliferation increases, malalignment and instability result. The changes are progressive, and C1–C2 and occipitocervical fusions are the surgical treatments of choice. These patients should be maintained in a cervical collar until their instability is treated.

Cervical spine involvement is present in 80% of patients who have had rheumatoid arthritis for over 10 years, and they should be screened for instability. Patients with more severe disease usually have cervical spine pathology. The following criteria are barometers for disease severity: female, high rheumatoid factor, younger age at diagnosis, rheumatoid nodules, non-drug-related eosinophilia, thrombocytosis, elevated C-reactive protein, and human leukocyte antigen (HLA)–DR4 genes.

In this case, the patient had advanced systemic disease and a poor quality of life. She and her family decided not to proceed with surgical treatment.

SUGGESTED READING

Nguyen HV, Ludwig SC, Silber J, et al. Rheumatoid arthritis of the cervical spine. Spine J 2004;4:329–334

19

Rheumatoid Patient with Ventral Cord Compression

■ Presentation

An 81-year-old man with a history of rheumatoid arthritis became progressively quadriparetic. He also complained of neck pain. On examination his motor strength was 3/5 in all of his extremities.

■ Radiologic Findings

Sagittal magnetic resonance imaging (MRI) of the cervical spine demonstrates a large, compressive pannus as well as subaxial spondylosis (**Fig. 19–1**).

■ Diagnosis

Pannus

■ Treatment

Occipitocervical stabilization was performed.

■ Discussion

Rheumatoid arthritis causes synovial inflammation, ligamentous laxity, and osseous erosion. All of this joint destruction causes micromotion at the occipitoatlantoaxial region, which can result in pannus formation. The pannus itself can compress the cervicomedullary junction, resulting in lower cranial nerve palsies, weakness, and myelopathy.

In this case, while the pannus is dramatic, its degree of cord compression is not. If it had been significantly compressive, a transoral route can be employed for ventral decompression of the cervicomedullary junction. Then the patient can be stabilized with a posterior instrumented fusion, usually from the occiput down to the subaxial spine. It is important to consider subaxial stability when deciding to which level the fusion should

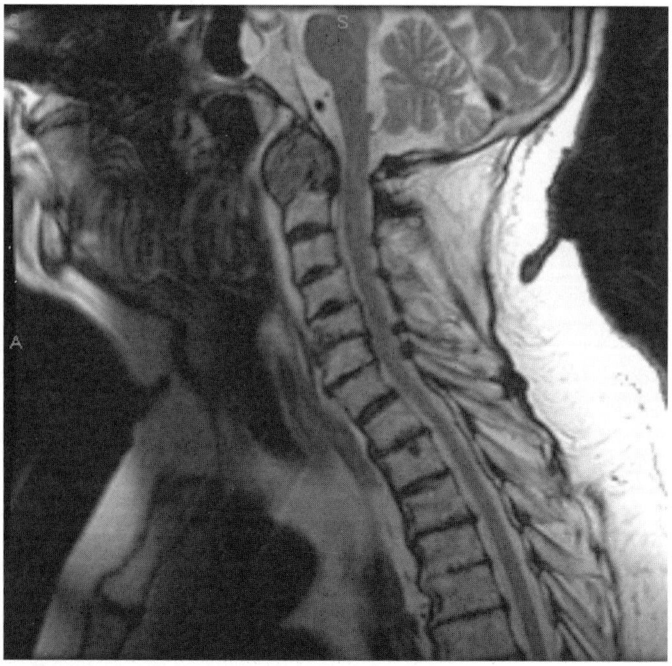

FIGURE 19–1 Sagittal MRI of the cervical spine demonstrates a large, compressive pannus as well as subaxial spondylosis.

be anchored. These patients' ligamentous laxity and degenerative disease of the spine can encompass multiple levels, and dynamic x-rays should be employed in their investigation.

SUGGESTED READING

Reijnierse M, Bloem JL, Dijkmans BA, et al. The cervical spine in rheumatoid arthritis: relationship between neurological signs and morphology of MR imaging and radiographs. Skeletal Radiol 1996;25:113–118

20

Rheumatoid Arthritis with Instability

■ Presentation

A 62-year-old woman with a history of rheumatoid arthritis developed progressive hoarseness and difficulty with swallowing. On examination she had lower cranial nerve palsies and hyperreflexia.

■ Radiologic Findings

Sagittal T2-weighted magnetic resonance imaging (MRI) and x-rays of the cervical spine show evidence of atlantoaxial instability, cord compression from a pannus and C1, and cord signal change at C1 (**Figs. 20–1** and **20–2**).

■ Diagnosis

Atlantoaxial instability and compression from rheumatoid changes

■ Treatment

A cervical decompression, reduction, and fusion from C0 (occiput) to C3 was performed (**Fig. 20–3**, lateral cervical x-ray).

■ Discussion

Rheumatoid patients commonly have neck pain, but only about a third have neurologic deficit. Of the cervical spine involvement, atlantoaxial instability is the most common and is due to an erosive synovitis that is part of the rheumatoid disease process. Pannus formation is due to the micromotion that occurs with ligamentous laxity.

The patient who is neurologically intact can usually be watched for progressive atlantodental interval increase (over 8 mm) or platybasia before surgery is warranted. But if the patient shows signs of cervicomedullary compression, a surgery to decompress and stabilize is needed. Rheumatoid patients are a high-risk surgical population because of their degree of systemic illness and long-term use of steroids and other anti-inflammatory medication.

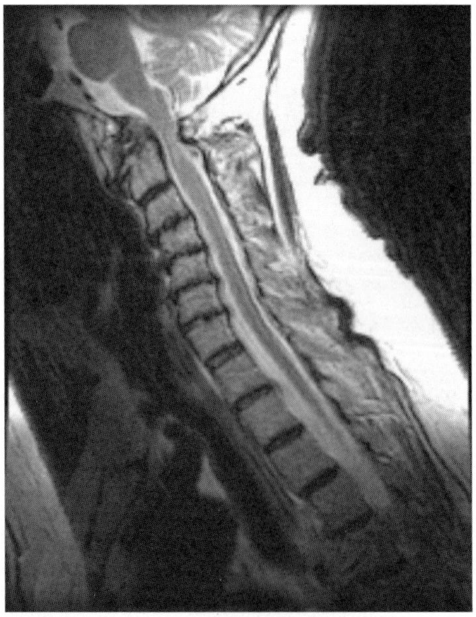

FIGURE 20–1 Sagittal MRI of the cervical spine shows a pannus, C1 compression, vertical migration of the dens, and cord signal change—all pathologies seen in rheumatoid arthritis patients with atlantoaxial subluxation.

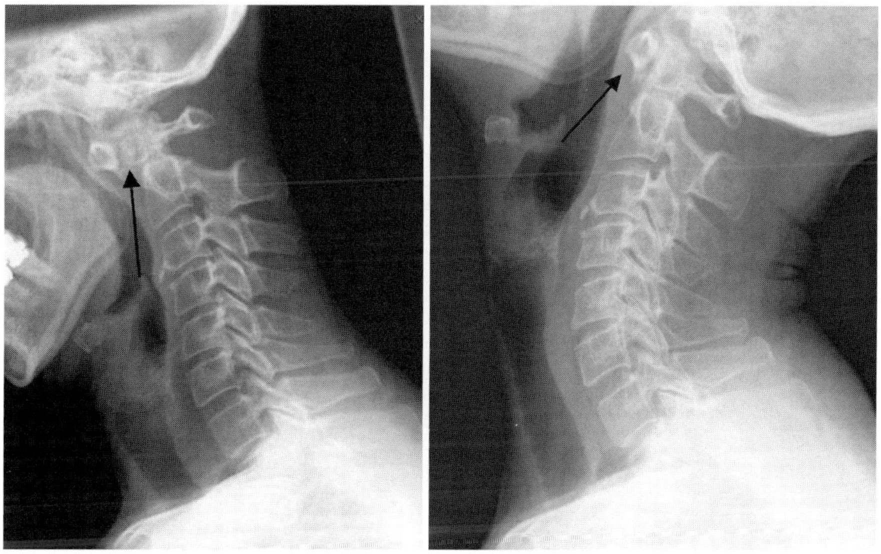

FIGURE 20–2 Flexion-extension cervical spine x-rays show an atlantodental interval of 9 mm on flexion, reducing on extension.

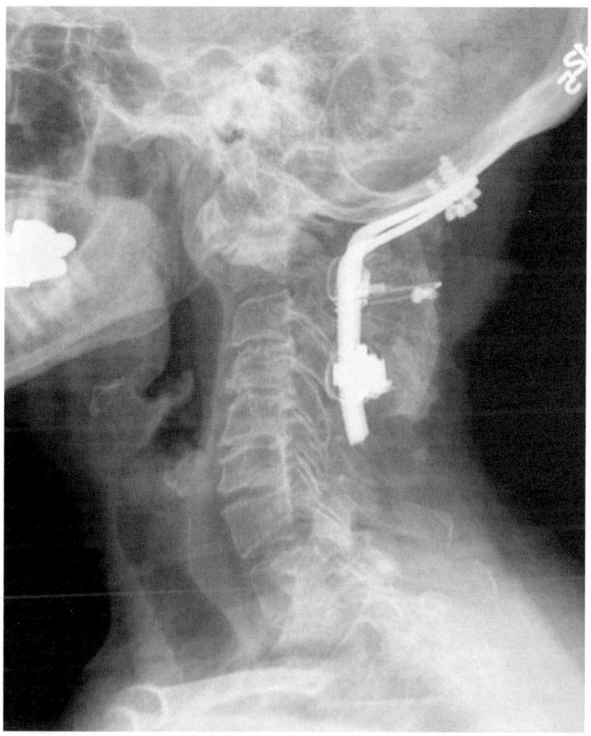

FIGURE 20–3 Postoperative hook-and-claw construct.

SUGGESTED READING

Nguyen HV, Ludwig SC, Silber J, et al. Rheumatoid arthritis of the cervical spine. Spine J 2004;4:329–334

herniation. It has many advantages over the anterior approach. Because it is less involved, it requires no fusion, which preserves the motion segment and decreases adjacent level disease. On the other hand, it is riskier and probably carries higher rate of recurrence. It is employed under the following conditions:

1. Unilateral pathology with the apex of the herniation lateral to the lateral margin of the cord
2. Absence of calcified disc or significant osteophyte
3. Absence of significant spondylosis or chronic axial neck pain, or radiographic evidence of mechanical instability
4. Absence of central stenosis
5. A professional singer or a professional in whom any chance of recurrent laryngeal nerve compromise is intolerable

A posterior laminotomy and foraminotomy can now be done percutaneously with a minimally invasive technique, less muscle dissection, and minimum blood loss. This fosters postoperative recovery and rehabilitation, with better functional status results. Several retractor systems have been designed for this purpose. In this case, the multilevel pathology was successfully addressed percutaneously. An anterior approach would have involved a multilevel fusion.

SUGGESTED READING

Russell SM, Benjamin V. Posterior surgical approach to the cervical neural foramen for intervertebral disc disease. Neurosurgery 2004;54:662–665

22

Cervical Cages

■ Presentation

A 55-year-old man complained of neck pain and a left upper extremity radiculopathy. He is neurologically intact and has evidence of cervical spondylosis, mostly at C3–C4 and C4–C5.

■ Radiologic Findings

An intraoperative radiograph shows the titanium cages at C3–C4 and C5–C6 (**Fig. 22–1**).

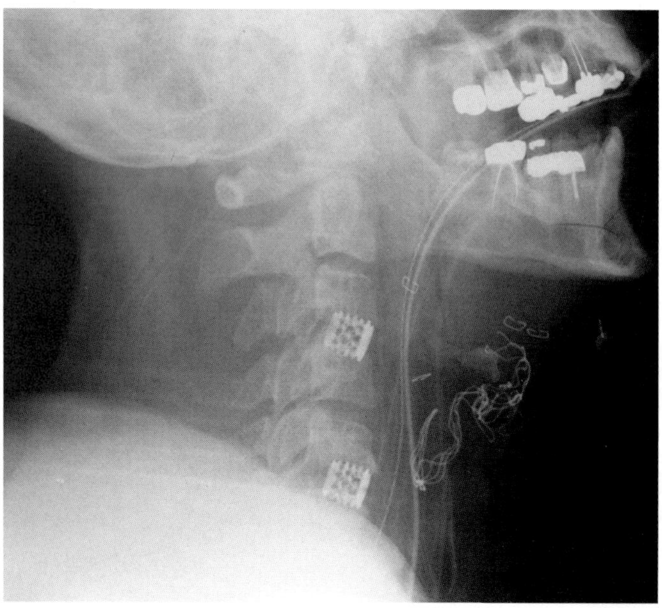

FIGURE 22–1 Intraoperative fluoroscopic image with titanium cages at C3–C4 and C5–C6.

■ Diagnosis

Cervical spondylosis with radiculopathy

■ Treatment

The patient underwent an anterior cervical discectomy and fusion with placement of autograft-filled threaded titanium cages at C3–C4 and C5–C6.

■ Discussion

Anterior cervical discectomy has been proven to be a safe and effective procedure for the treatment of degenerative disc disease. There are several options when performing multilevel anterior cervical decompressions, ranging from multiple discectomies to corpectomy with allograft or autograft. These procedures can be done with or without plating. More recently, titanium cage–augmented fusion with or without plate fixation has come into vogue.

Placement of interbody fusion cages can restore physiologic disc height, improve sagittal balance, and provide immediate load-bearing support. Unlike autograft and allograft, cages are not associated with implant collapse even when assessed 1 year following surgery. These interbody devices facilitate interbody arthrodesis, and prevent donor-site morbidity. Interbody cages are called "no profile internal fixation" because they provide immediate segmental stabilization by tensing the ligamentous apparatus, while avoiding plate-related morbidities. Such complications include esophageal complications, hoarseness, and other hardware-related failure.

With the recent introduction of motion preservation technology, this patient may prove to be a good candidate for cervical disc arthroplasty, especially with the presence of tandem disc disease and a relatively normal intervening segment. This new technology is introduced to maintain motion and potentially minimize adjacent segment degeneration. However, typical to any new technology, there are some drawbacks. The need for longer follow-up studies, artificial disc retrieval, and procedural learning curves are some of the negatives.

SUGGESTED READINGS

Hacker RJ. Threaded cages for degenerative cervical disease. Clin Orthop 2002;394:39–46

Hwang SL, Lin CL, Lieu AS, et al. Three-level and four-level anterior cervical discectomies and titanium cage-augmented fusion with and without plate fixation. J Neurosurg Spine 2004;1:160–167

23

Mechanical Neck Pain

Presentation

A 41-year-old woman began complaining of neck pain, with some radicular component, after a car accident. It had been interrupting her life for months and had not responded to physical therapy. She was neurologically intact. Magnetic resonance imaging (MRI) of the cervical spine demonstrated degenerative spine disease, mostly at C3–C4 and C4–C5, with ventral cord compression and reversal of the normal cervical lordosis.

Radiologic Findings

The postoperative construct of a C4 corpectomy with allograft fusion and plate on a lateral cervical x-ray is shown in **Fig. 23–1**.

Diagnosis

Cervical spondylitic disease

Treatment

C4 corpectomy with allograft fusion

Discussion

Degenerative cervical spine disease can be a source of neck pain that can be disabling at times. In a carefully selected patient who has failed all other noninvasive modalities of treatment, a cervical fusion can eliminate the pain generator.

Cervical fusion surgery can be done anteriorly or posteriorly. The anterior approach addresses the ventral elements, eliminates micromotion, and can create a successful fusion result. In this case, the patient's pain improved postoperatively.

SUGGESTED READING

Ferch RD, Shad A, Cadoux-Hudson TA, Teddy PJ. Anterior correction of cervical kyphotic deformity: effects on myelopathy, neck pain, and sagittal alignment. J Neurosurg 2004;100(1 Suppl Spine): 13–19

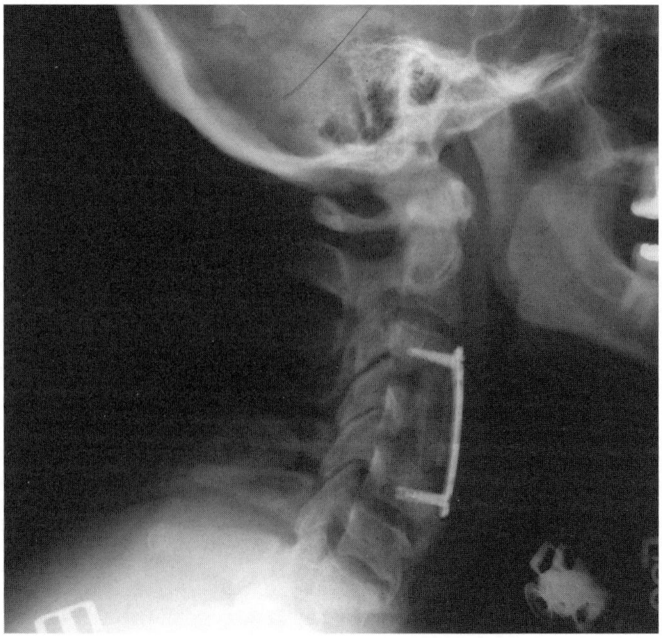

FIGURE 23–1 C4 corpectomy with allograft fusion and plate.

24

Multilevel Anterior Cervical Discectomy and Fusion (ACDF)

■ Presentation

A 52-year-old woman with neck pain and myelopathy had a progressive swan neck deformity.

■ Radiologic Findings

Abnormal cervical kyphosis is evident on sagittal C-spine magnetic resonance imaging (MRI) (**Fig. 24–1**).

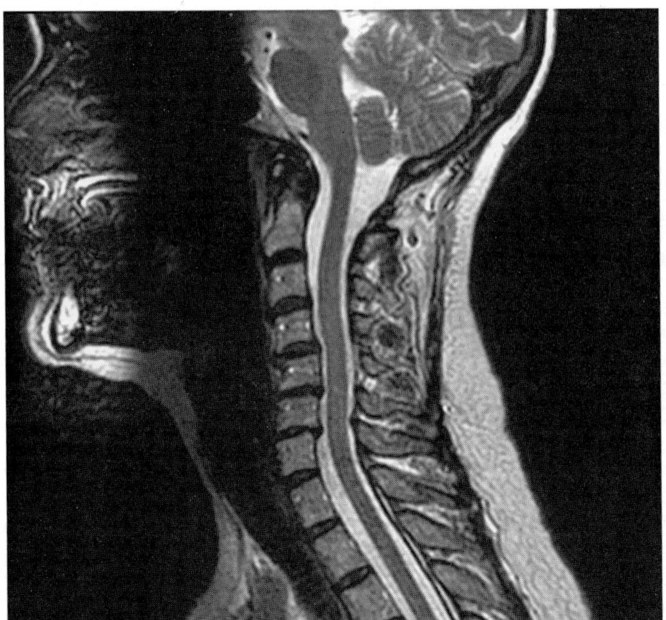

FIGURE 24–1 Abnormal cervical kyphosis on sagittal C-spine MRI.

■ Diagnosis

Degenerative cervical subluxation

■ Treatment

A multilevel anterior cervical discectomy and fusion (ACDF) was completed, along with reintroduction of cervical lordosis. This is seen on postoperative lateral cervical x-ray (**Fig. 24–2**).

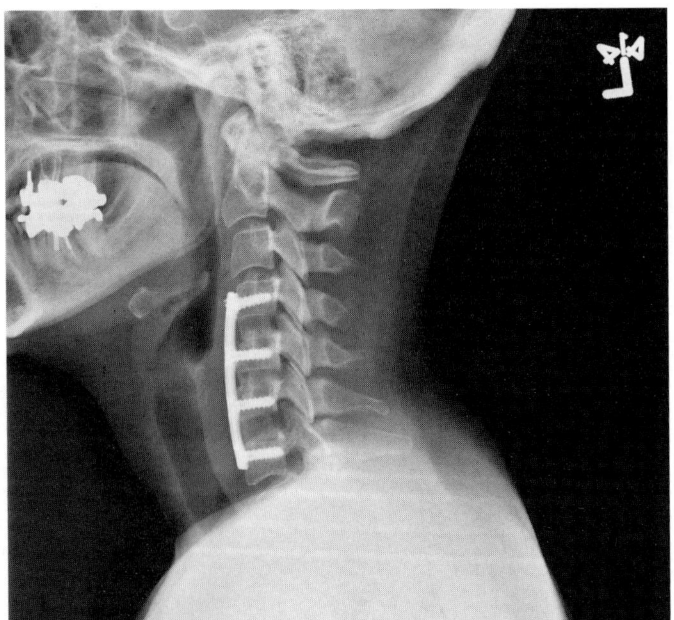

FIGURE 24–2 Reintroduction of cervical lordosis through multilevel ACDF as imaged on x-ray.

■ Discussion

Cervical kyphosis can be degenerative, congenital, compensatory, posttraumatic, or iatrogenic. Usually it is associated with myelopathy. The normal cervical lordotic curve is 15 to 20 degrees from C1 to T1. Straightening of this curve increases with age as disc height loss becomes more evident. Cervical kyphosis is a kyphotic angulation of 5 degrees or more.

Certain considerations should be given when planning a multilevel ACDF. There is a 10-degree loss of cervical motion for each fused motion segment. Adjacent level disc degeneration is more common after a multilevel procedure and is usually the rostral space. The rate of pseudarthrosis increases with each level fused. Dysphagia rates increase as well.

Anterior decompression and grafting is the preferred approach when dealing with cervical kyphosis. If there is significant posterior compression with spondylitic changes, a combined anterior-posterior decompression and fusion is needed. Re-creation of cervical lordosis through a multilevel ACDF can decelerate adjacent segment degeneration. Cervical lordosis in this case was re-created by securing the most rostral and caudal screws in the screw/plate construct. Then "salvage" screws were introduced into the two mid-construct vertebral bodies and carefully tightened to bring the middle subluxed vertebrae into sagittal realignment.

SUGGESTED READING

Samartzis D, Shen FH, Matthews DK, Yoon ST, Goldberg EJ, An HS. Comparison of allograft to autograft in multilevel anterior cervical discectomy and fusion with rigid plate fixation. Spine J 2003; 3:451–459

25

Hardware Failure

■ Presentation

A 38-year-old woman had an earlier C3–C4 anterior cervical discectomy and fusion. She continued to complain of neck pain. Workup demonstrated hardware failure; the upper and lower screws had backed out.

■ Radiologic Findings

Lateral cervical x-ray revealed the previously placed C3 and C4 screws had backed out along with the plate, and the allograft had resorbed (**Fig. 25–1**).

■ Diagnosis

Cervical pseudarthrosis

■ Treatment

The patient underwent laryngoscopic evaluation to ensure there was no subclinical unilateral recurrent laryngeal nerve palsy. Then she had a contralateral anterior cervical approach to retrieve the failing hardware, followed by posterior C3–C5 lateral mass fusion with autograft.

■ Discussion

The most common form of hardware failure after anterior cervical plating is screw back-out. Nonunion in this region usually has this presentation. Another common reason for this occurrence is placement of the screws adjacent to or through the end plate. Risks of cervical nonunion include smoking, use of allograft in a multilevel fusion in a smoker, nonsteroidal anti-inflammatory drug (NSAID) use, and noncompliance with external orthosis in the postoperative period.

When performing a reoperation for hardware failure, ideally one wants to avoid a scarred dissection. Laryngoscopic evaluation is needed to ensure that there is no subclinical unilateral recurrent laryngeal nerve palsy. This palsy could potentially lead to fatal postoperative upper airway obstruction. In addition, a contralateral

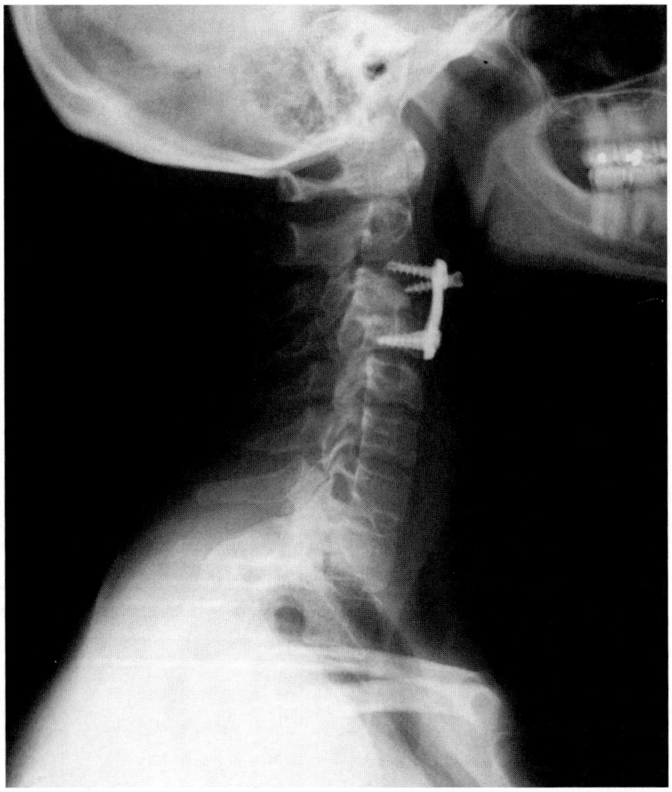

FIGURE 25–1 Pseudoarthrosis is seen at C3–C4 with hardware failure.

approach through scarless tissue lowers operative morbidity. Here, an anterior approach was used to retrieve the failing hardware, and the spine was then stabilized posteriorly with good result.

SUGGESTED READING

Herrmann AM, Geisler FH. Geometric results of anterior cervical plate stabilization in degenerative disease. Spine 2004;29: 1226–1234

26

Postoperative Kyphosis

■ Presentation

A 47-year-old woman underwent a previous C4 corpectomy for cervicomyeloradiculopathy. Her extant swan neck deformity and symptoms worsened postoperatively.

■ Radiologic Findings

Preoperatively, the patient had cervical stenosis and kyphosis (**Fig. 26–1**). After a C4 corpectomy, her kyphosis increased, as exhibited on T2-weighted sagittal cervical magnetic resonance imaging (MRI) and sagittal cervical computed tomography (CT) reconstruction (**Figs. 26–2** and **26–3**).

■ Diagnosis

Iatrogenic instability

■ Treatment

Revision and extension of her previous anterior cervical corpectomy and fusion with lateral mass plating posteriorly was undertaken (**Fig. 26–4**).

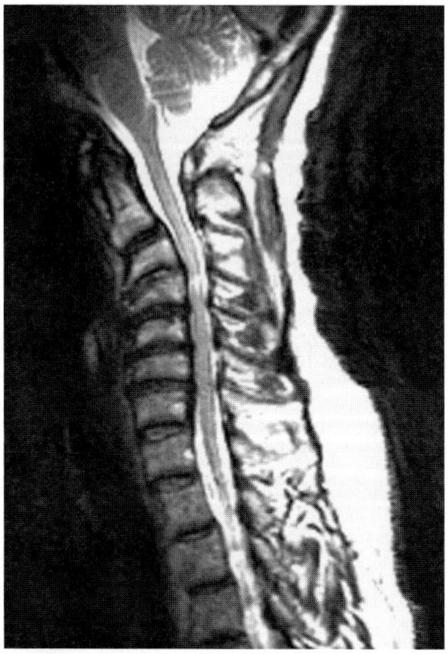

FIGURE 26–1 Preoperative cervical MRI with severe cervical spondylosis.

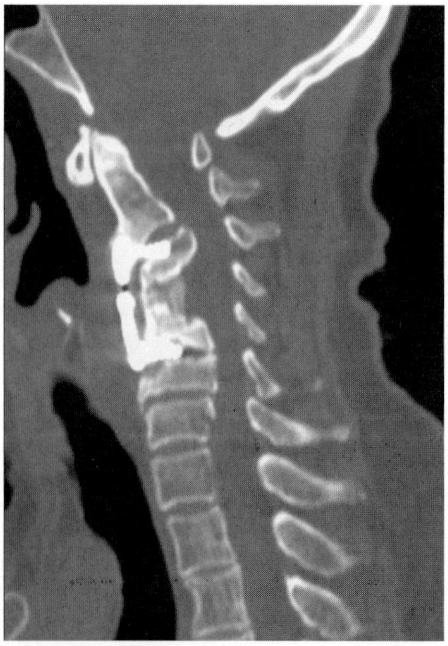

FIGURE 26–2 Failure of the construct as seen on CT scan of the cervical spine.

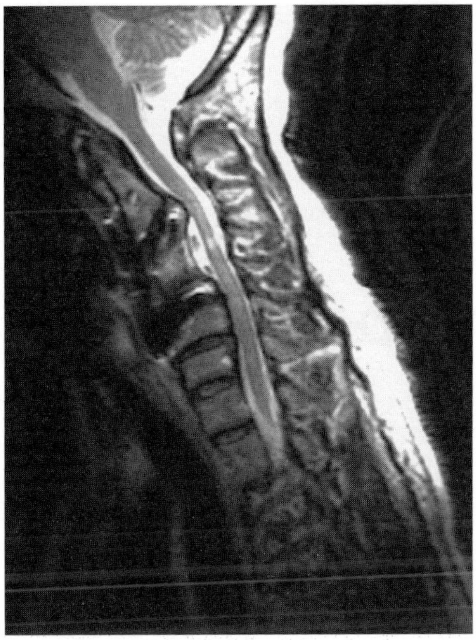

FIGURE 26–3 MRI of the cervical spine showing accelerated postoperative kyphosis.

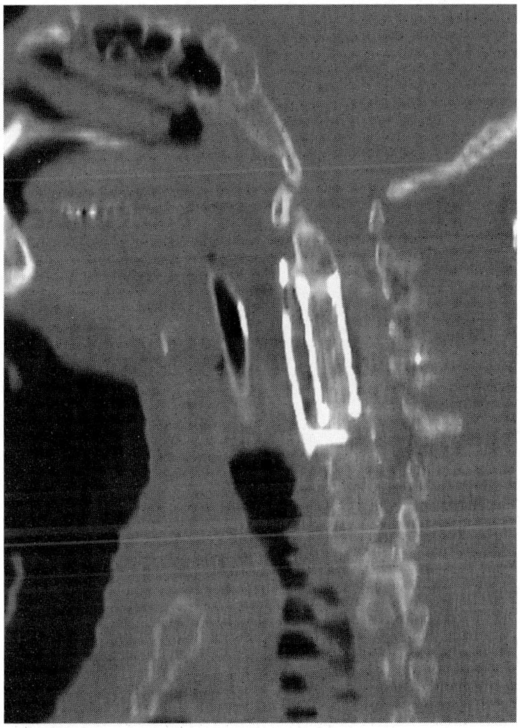

FIGURE 26–4 Revision construct.

■ Discussion

In determining which approach is suitable for the cervical spine, consider the spine contour and etiology of the pathology. Failure to address the full picture will lead to pseudarthrosis. One needs to understand the mechanics of plating. Place the screws away from the adjacent end plate or disc space, as misplacement will accelerate adjacent level disease. To fully reintroduce cervical lordosis, the plate may need to be contoured. If the patient has a multilevel pathology with cervical kyphosis, a 360-degree fusion may be necessary.

In cases of pseudarthrosis, hardware failure is often the first manifestation. This is more common with allograft. Pain, kyphosis, screw back-out, and myelopathy are other signs. Revision surgery is more risky, and one may elect to go posteriorly as a salvage approach. In this case, the patient's ventral column support was inadequate, so we had to fuse her anteriorly and posteriorly. A three-level anterior corpectomy with a titanium cage reconstruction, autograft, and supplemental posterior tension band from C2–C7 was done.

The question sometimes arises regarding the caudal extent of the fusion. We stopped just above the cervicothoracic junction, although the spinal orientation changes here. The patient was young and had a multilevel fixation and a normal cervicothoracic junction. Thus we did not incorporate T1 or T2, but she should be watched for possible future degeneration. Additionally, intraoperative judgment plays a role in refining the preoperative plan according to electrophysiologic monitoring data and findings of instability. One should be cautious to avoid a dural tear and not to overdistract the spine. Revision cases always have an added complexity.

SUGGESTED READING

Steinmetz MP, Kager CD, Benzel EC. Ventral correction of postsurgical cervical kyphosis. J Neurosurg 2003;98:1–7

27

Multilevel Cervical Stenosis

■ Presentation

A 53-year-old woman with a history of cervical discectomy presented with progressive neck pain, spasticity, and hand clumsiness. She was myelopathic and had mild left upper extremity weakness. Her magnetic resonance imaging (MRI) revealed marked cervical spondylosis with anterior cord compression at C2–C3, C4–C5, and C5–C6.

■ Radiologic Findings

A three-level corpectomy with fibular strut graft and buttress plate is shown on postoperative computed tomography (CT) of the cervical spine with sagittal reconstruction (**Fig. 27–1**).

■ Diagnosis

Cervical spondylitic myelopathy

■ Treatment

Anterior C3–C5 corpectomies with fibular graft, arthrodesis, and buttress plate, and then a posterior C2–C6 instrumented arthrodesis and autograft were done.

■ Discussion

Cervical stenosis can be addressed in multiple ways. In this case, the cord compression is anterior and multileveled. A C3–C5 corpectomy with fibular graft arthrodesis and instrumentation would directly address the patient's pathology, whereas a multilevel posterior cervical decompression would be less effective. The addition of posterior instrumentation following a multilevel corpectomy tends to create a solid fixation and reduces the chance of nonunion and hardware failure. Thin-cut CT scan of the neck with sagittal reformatting was used for preoperative planning.

Also, the patient was seen by an ear, nose, and throat specialist to clear her of possible subclinical recurrent laryngeal nerve injury, as this was the patient's second

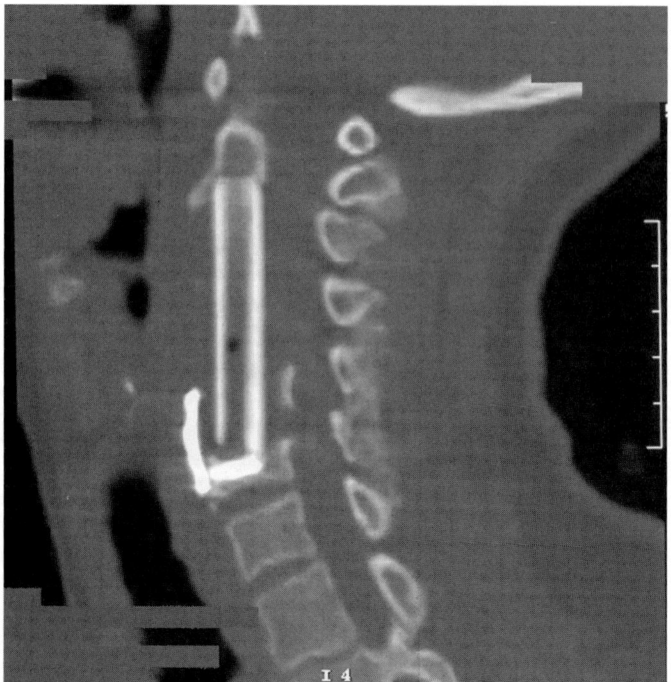

FIGURE 27–1 The anterior construct, with fibular graft and buttress plate, is shown on CT reconstruction.

anterior approach to the cervical spine, this time from the opposing side. Because of the nature of redo anterior neck dissections, patients need to be screened for subclinical recurrent laryngeal nerve injury.

SUGGESTED READING

Beutler WJ, Sweeney CA, Connolly PJ. Recurrent laryngeal nerve injury with anterior cervical spine surgery risk with laterality of surgical approach. Spine 2001;26:1337–1342

28

Ossification of the Posterior Longitudinal Ligament (OPLL)

■ Presentation

A 77-year-old Asian man fell, sustaining a central cord syndrome. His neurologic functioning improved except for some fine motor difficulty and continued myelopathy. After rehabilitation, he returned for operative planning.

■ Radiologic Findings

Magnetic resonance imaging (MRI) of the cervical spine (**Figs. 28–1** and **28–2**) shows cervical stenosis, most significantly at C5 and C6, with ossification of the posterior longitudinal ligament (OPLL) and cord signal change.

■ Diagnosis

Cervical stenosis with OPLL and cord signal change

■ Treatment

An anterior cervical decompression and fusion was accomplished.

■ Discussion

Ossification of the posterior longitudinal ligament, although typically seen in Japanese patients, can be associated with degenerative disease, diabetes, or ankylosing spondylitis. The posterior longitudinal ligament undergoes some combination of hypertrophy, ossification, and calcification. It can appear in separate segments, as a continual band, or as a mixture. Patients present with myeloradicular symptoms or central cord syndrome after a fall.

Treatment options vary. Extensive literature has documented a variety of laminoplasty techniques. The posterior approach has the benefit of avoiding the pathology

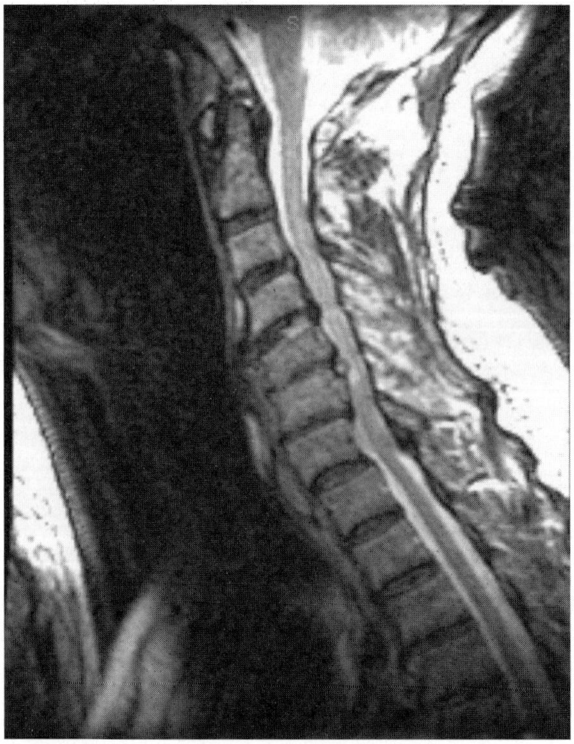

FIGURE 28–1 Sagittal T2-weighted MRI of the cervical spine shows severe cervical spondylitic disease, most prominently at C5 and C6. In addition, segmental OPLL is seen.

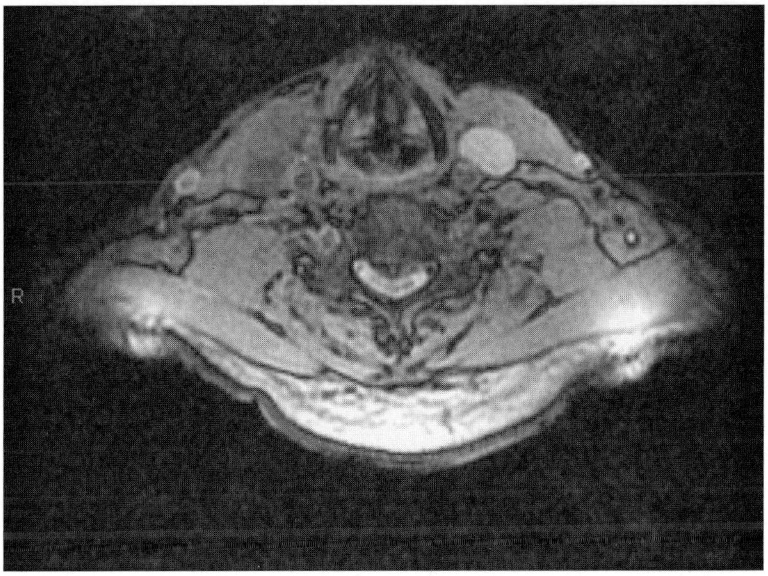

FIGURE 28–2 Axial cut of a cervical MRI displays the typical ventral ossification noted in OPLL.

while providing room for the cervical cord. The anterior approach directly addresses the pathology but has a higher risk of unintended durotomy and possible neurologic damage. Neurophysiologic monitoring during the case is a worthwhile consideration.

In this case, ventral decompression was selected to address the patient's notable amount of ventral compression. A fiberoptic intubation was done. Intraoperatively, the dura was adherent and compressed by the posterior longitudinal ligament (PLL), but was freed. The patient achieved a solid fusion and was able to return to his previous level of activity.

SUGGESTED READING

Matsunaga S, Sakou T, Taketomi E, Komiya S. Clinical course of patients with ossification of the posterior longitudinal ligament: a minimum 10 year cohort study. J Neurosurg 2004;100(3 Suppl Spine):245–248

29

Cervical Myelopathy

■ Presentation

A 44-year-old man with chronic neck pain began experiencing hand numbness. On examination he was myelopathic.

■ Radiologic Findings

A T2-weighted sagittal magnetic resonance imaging (MRI) of the cervical spine revealed C3 through C6 ventral cord compression (**Fig. 29–1**).

■ Diagnosis

Cervical spondylomyelopathy

■ Treatment

A 360-degree cervical fusion, with a three-level corpectomy, titanium cage, and plating anteriorly, and a lateral mass fixation posteriorly (**Figs. 29–2** and **29–3**) were done.

■ Discussion

Several factors are considered in determining surgical approach when faced with cervical spondylomyelopathy. These include cervical contour, presence or absence of kyphosis, the nature and length of the compression, the patient's overall condition and bone quality, and the surgeon's experience with a given approach. This patient presented with significant myelopathy at a relatively young age. Because of his ventral cord compression, a multilevel corpectomy was needed to sufficiently decompress the cord.

There are several long-arm corpectomy graft options. Autograft is a safe and successful option, but obtaining one to fit a three-level corpectomy can be challenging. A structural fibular allograft is another option, but this takes a long time (up to 2 years) to incorporate, hence increasing

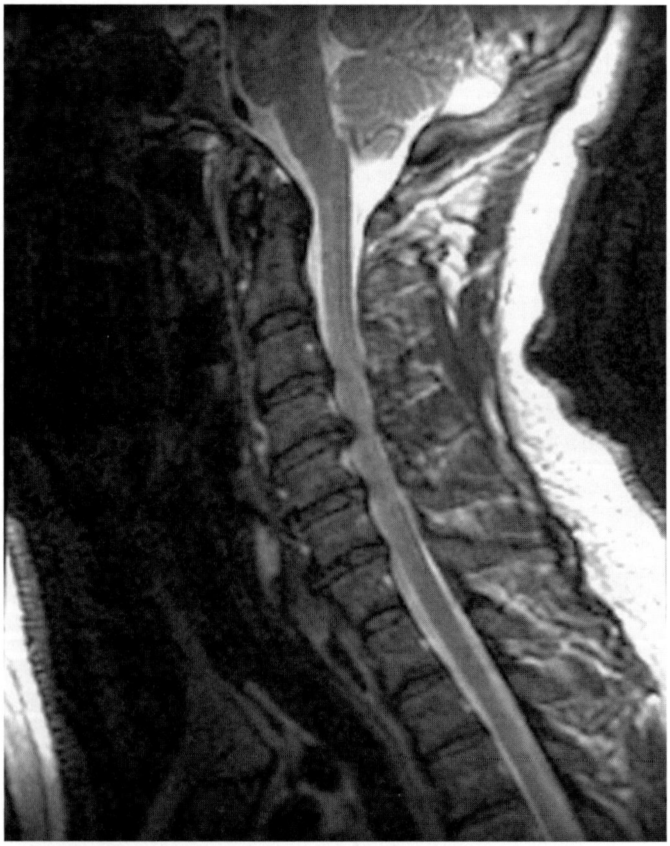

FIGURE 29–1 MRI of the cervical spine with significant degenerative disc disease.

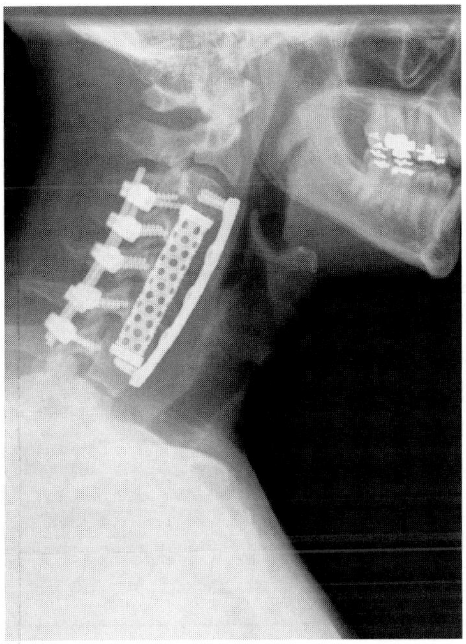

FIGURE 29–2 Postoperative lateral C-spine x-ray demonstrating the 360-degree construct, featuring a three-level titanium cage.

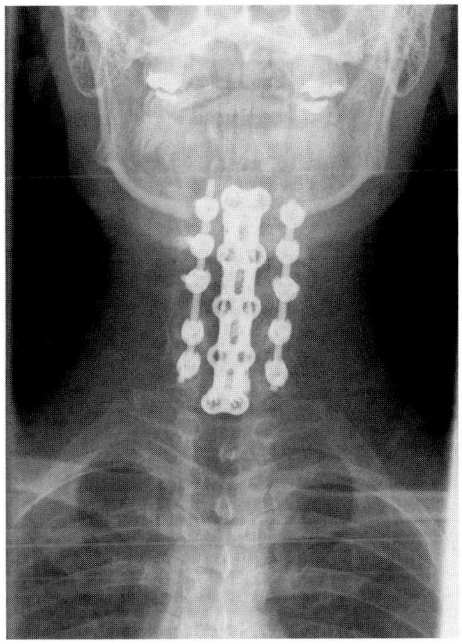

FIGURE 29–3 Postoperative anterior-posterior cervical x-ray with the postoperative construct.

the chances of pseudarthrosis. An alternative method is the use of titanium cage packed with one of many possible bone graft materials. The core space of the cage becomes the center of the final arthrodesis. The use of bone morphogenetic protein has been gaining popularity. It enhances arthrodesis, but in this location is an off-label use and carries a significant potential for morbidity.

SUGGESTED READING

Anderson DG, Albert TJ. Bone grafting, implants, and plating options for anterior cervical fusions. Orthop Clin North Am 2002; 33:317–328

30

Cervical Hardware Failure

■ Presentation

A 55-year-old woman previously underwent a multilevel corpectomy for cervical stenosis and now presents with hardware failure.

■ Radiologic Findings

Cervical x-ray and myelogram computed tomography (CT) (**Figs. 30–1** and **30–2**) display a cervical fusion construct with ventrocaudal extrusion of the cage and plate.

■ Diagnosis

Hardware "kick out"

■ Treatment

After traction to reduce her anterior subluxation, plate removal and case repositioning was done. Structural autograft was inserted at C7–T1, and posterior C2–T1 segmental fusion with autograft completed the case.

■ Discussion

After an ear, nose, and throat (ENT) evaluation to determine vocal cord veracity in preparation for an opposite-side cervical approach to avoid previous scar, the patient underwent a 360-degree cervical fusion. The support of a sound postoperative external orthosis will increase her chances of successful arthrodesis. She wore a pinless halo

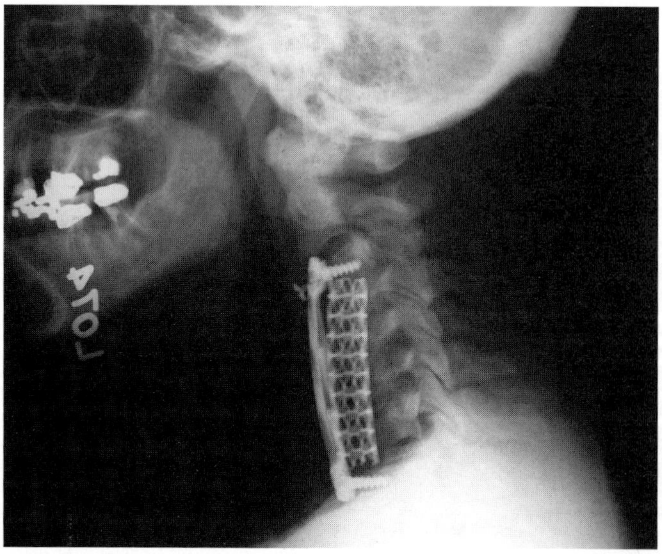

FIGURE 30–1 Lateral cervical x-ray with ventrocaudal "kick out" of the construct.

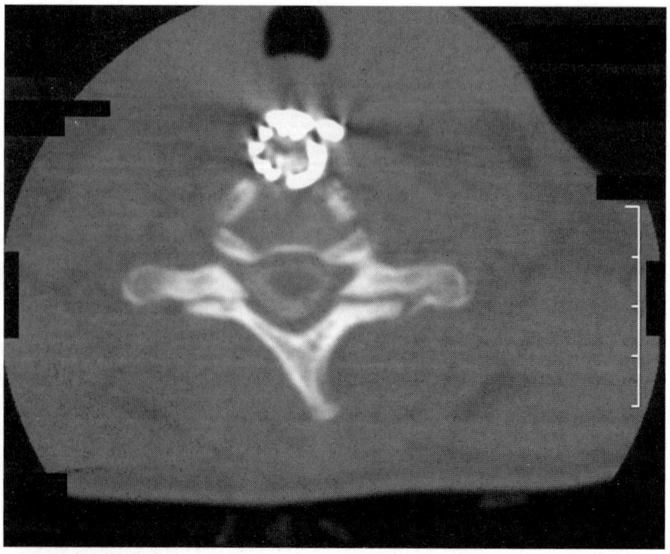

FIGURE 30–2 CT myelogram again showing hardware failure.

for 4 months after surgery and was given an external bone stimulator. She also stopped smoking. All of these items will enhance results in a redo patient. Nonunion and cage malposition provide for a challenging redo surgery. The cage can scar in, creating a high morbidity risk. In this case, we were able to free the cage enough to reposition it. Also, the anterior fusion was supplemented through the addition of a posterior tension band with posterolateral arthrodesis.

SUGGESTED READING

Wang JC, Hart RA, Emery SE, Bohlman HH. Graft migration or displacement after multilevel cervical corpectomy and strut grafting. Spine 2003;28:1016–1021

31

Central Cord with Osteoporosis

■ Presentation

A 79-year-old woman sustained central cord syndrome after a fall, with significant upper extremity weakness and incontinence. She had multilevel cervical disc herniations and concomitant osteoporosis. Magnetic resonance imaging (MRI) showed cervical spondylosis with a large soft herniated disc at C4–C5 and cord signal change. Due to progressive neurologic deterioration, the decision was made to treat her surgically.

■ Radiologic Findings

Postoperative lateral cervical x-ray displays a fibular strut graft spanning from C3 to C6 with a buttress plate and significant osteopenia (**Fig. 31–1**).

■ Diagnosis

Central cord syndrome with acute disc

■ Treatment

An anterior cervical discectomy at C3–C4 and C5–C6, with C4 and C5 corpectomies, and reconstruction with a fibular strut graft, arthrodesis, and buttress plate were completed.

■ Discussion

Central cord syndrome is a partial neurologic deficit, with motor more than sensory loss, upper more than lower extremity deficit, and distal more than proximal involvement. Pathologically, one sees a significant cord contusion. Acute decompression has been thought to carry a higher neurologic morbidity, and surgery is usually performed on a delayed, elective basis. If signs of progressive neurologic deterioration are apparent, then acute decompression is warranted. Also, if the patient has an acute disc herniation or findings suggesting instability, such as dislocation, more urgent surgical intervention may be warranted. This patient had the neurologic indications for surgery but carried a high risk of nonunion due to her age, osteoporosis, and multilevel fusion. She wore a cervical collar for 3 months

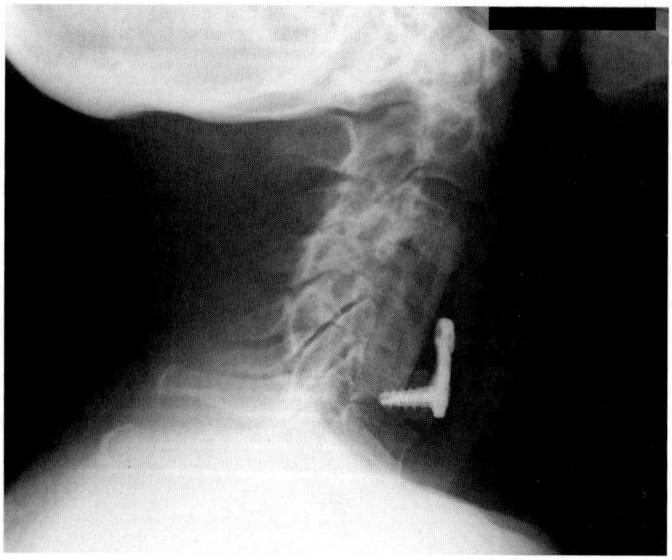

FIGURE 31–1 Postoperative cervical x-ray reveals a corpectomy fusion mass and buttress plate.

after surgery and was given a cervical bone stimulator. Her recovery went well, with resolution of the incontinence and improvement of her upper extremity strength.

SUGGESTED READING

Guest J, Eleraky MA, Apostolides PJ, Dickman CA, Sonntag VK. Traumatic central cord syndrome: results of surgical management. J Neurosurg 2002;97:25–32

32

Pseudomeningocele

■ Presentation

An 82-year-old man presents with a cervical pseudomeningocele, discovered 2 years after multilevel posterior cervical laminectomy. Neurologically, he has been stable. He has a significant cardiopulmonary history.

■ Radiologic Findings

A cervical magnetic resonance imaging (MRI) demonstrates postsurgical changes from C2 to C7, as well as a large intradural fluid collection with cerebrospinal fluid (CSF) signal intensity in the operative bed (**Fig. 32–1**).

■ Diagnosis

Iatrogenic pseudomeningocele

■ Treatment

No treatment is needed.

■ Discussion

The patient is asymptomatic with an intact wound and stable neurologic status. His surgery was done 2 years ago, and he has significant medical comorbidities. In this case, there is no need for surgical intervention. If he had an active CSF leak or was experiencing cord compression, one might consider further investigation or surgical repair of this likely pseudomeningocele, all the while keeping in mind his medical history. Pseudomeningocele is not an uncommon occurrence following spine surgery in the elderly, particularly in redo cases. The use of power tools, such as the drill, has likely contributed to a higher frequency of this pathology. One needs to take meticulous care with dural closure in case of durotomy, using direct repair, fibrin glue, and a watertight fascial closure. The skin should be closed meticulously, and one may consider using interrupted vertical mattress sutures. The head of the bed should be elevated for the first

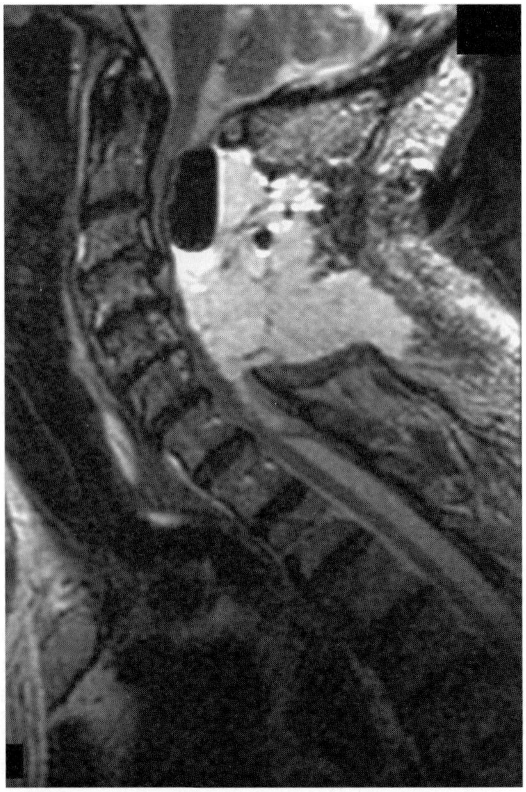

FIGURE 32–1 Sagittal cervical MRI with postoperative pseudomeningocele.

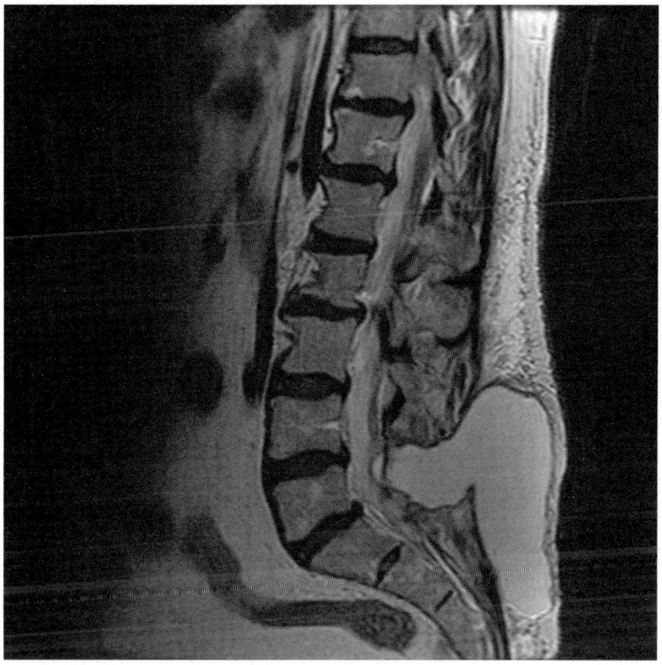

FIGURE 32–2 Sagittal lumbar MRI with a pseudomeningocele.

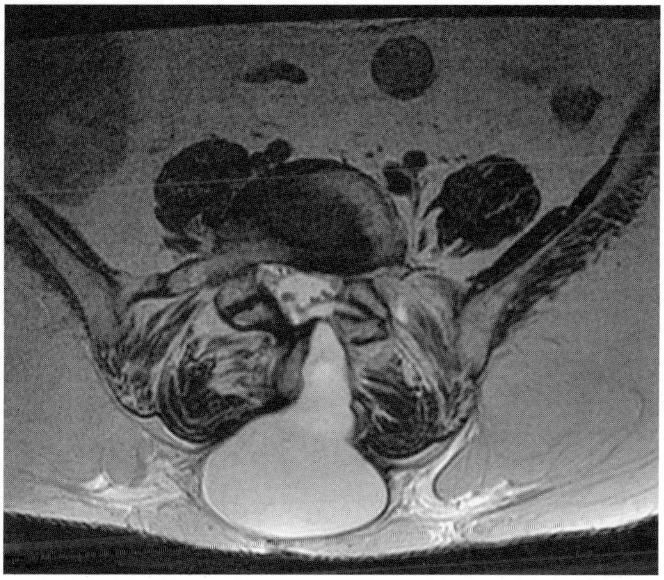

FIGURE 32–3 Axial lumbar MRI with a pseudomeningocele.

24 hours in the case of a cervical leak, and flat in the case of a lumbar leak (**Figs. 32–2** and **32–3**). The wound should be frequently checked, and patients need to be observed for signs of low-pressure headache. MRI and computed tomography (CT) myelogram are the imaging tests of choice. Revision surgery may be required.

SUGGESTED READING

Ross JS. Magnetic resonance imaging of the postoperative spine. Semin Musculoskel Radiol 2000;4:281–291

33

Angioedema

■ Presentation

A 29-year-old man with cervical myelopathy secondary to ventral cord compression underwent a two-level corpectomy and interbody fusion using a titanium cage and cervical plate. The cage had been packed with morselized autograft and small pieces of bone morphogenetic protein (BMP). Four days postoperatively he experienced stridor and severe airway swelling, necessitating emergency intubation.

■ Radiologic Findings

Soft tissue computed tomography (CT) of the neck shows left-sided soft tissue swelling with midline shift of the intubated airway (**Fig. 33–1**).

■ Diagnosis

Possible BMP-related angioedema

■ Treatment

The patient was kept intubated for a few days, until the airway swelling resolved.

■ Discussion

BMP is a recombinant technology that has been effective in inducing early osteoblast activity. It triggers a cascade of biologic events, including activating a series of inflammatory cell lines. There have been few reports of delayed but significant soft tissue swelling a few days following BMP use in anterior cervical procedures. The presentation resembles swelling from angioedema. Dysphagia, hoarseness, stridor, and airway compromise develop, and if not addressed, can be life threatening. This seems to occur on days 4 to 7 postoperatively. The timing is of some significance, because patients are usually going to be discharged or already at home by this time.

When confronted with these symptoms, emergent intubation by someone experienced in difficult airway management and high-dose steroids should be strongly considered. A steroid course is maintained while serial CT scans of the neck are done to assess for swelling resolution prior to extubation. The differential for the abovementioned constellation of symptoms encompasses more common complications, such as a postoperative

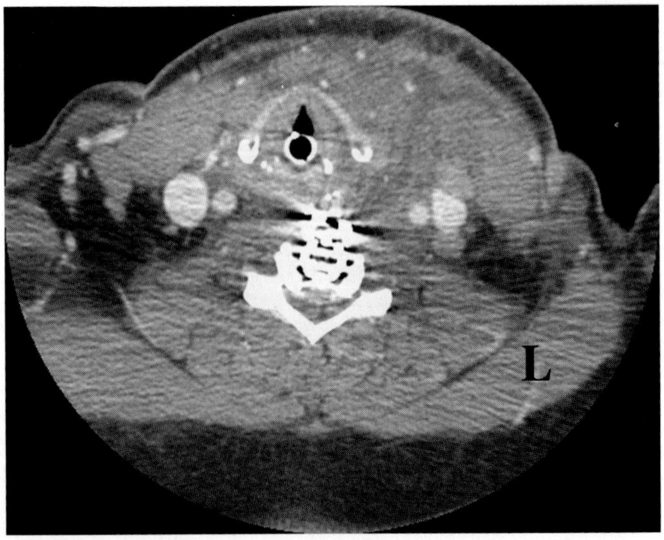

FIGURE 33–1 Notice the amount of swelling in the left sternocleidomastoid and surrounding tissue in comparison to the right side. There is over 1 cm of airway midline shift.

hematoma or infection. Certainly, a combination of tissue manipulation, the long duration of surgery, and the length of construct could all contribute to this patient's swelling.

We feel the use of BMP in anterior cervical procedures can be associated with some risk and is dose dependent. Only a small volume of the BMP sponge is required to induce the osteoblastic reaction required to enhance fusion. In the cervical spine, larger doses are of no additional benefit and may lead to a significant inflammatory response with morbid cervical swelling. Notably, it is not Food and Drug Administration (FDA) approved for this location. Additionally, BMP should be avoided in pregnant women, women planning a pregnancy in the subsequent 6 months, or in patients diagnosed with primary or secondary bone tumors.

SUGGESTED READING

Boakye M, Mummaneni PV, Garrett M, Rodts G, Haid R. Anterior cervical diskectomy and fusion involving a polyetheretherketone spacer and bone morphogenetic protein. J Neurosurg Spine 2005;2:521–525

■ SECTION B ■

Thoracic

34

Thoracic Disc

■ Presentation

A 60-year-old man presented with progressive paraplegia and a thoracic sensory level.

■ Radiologic Findings

A thoracic magnetic resonance imaging (MRI) showed a T8–T9 disc with thecal sac compression (**Figs. 34–1** and **34–2**).

■ Diagnosis

Thoracic disc extrusion with cord compression

■ Treatment

A thoracic laminectomy and pediculectomy was performed to gain access to the disc space for its removal.

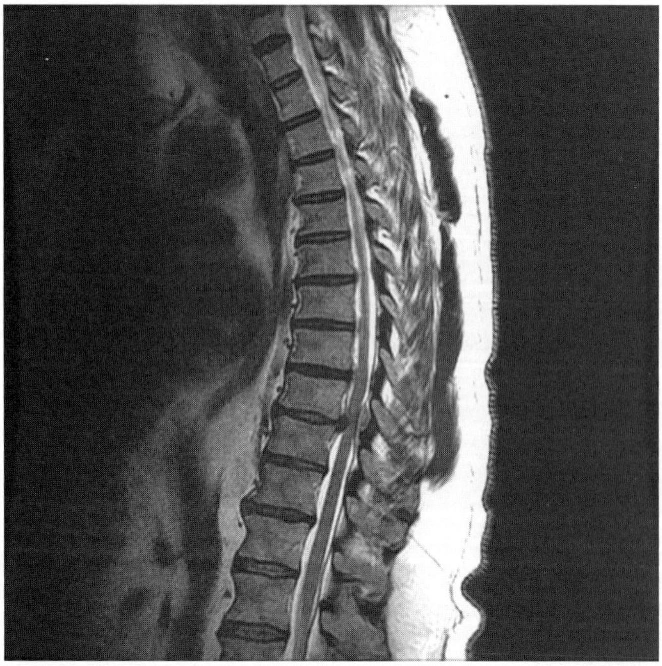

FIGURE 34–1 Sagittal thoracic T2-weighted MRI showing a thoracic disc protrusion compressing the cord.

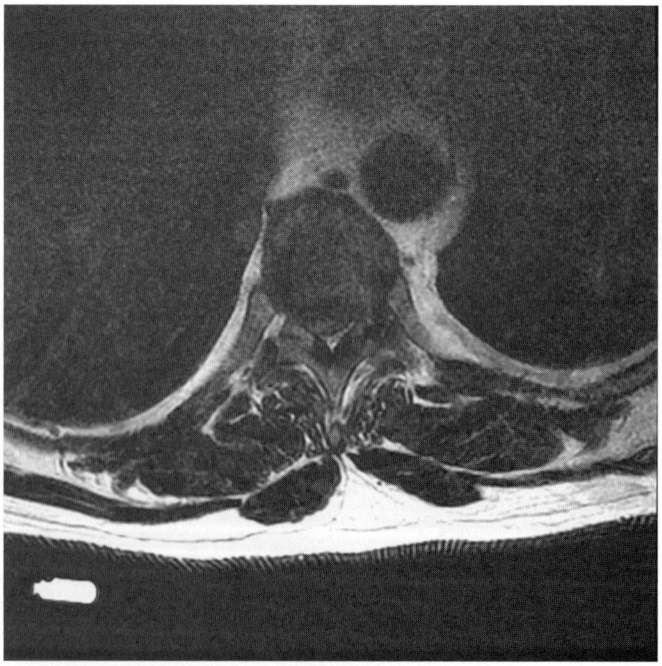

FIGURE 34–2 Axial T2-weighted thoracic MRI demonstrating the circumferential cord compression.

TABLE 36–1 Intramedullary Spinal Cord Lesion Differential

Degenerative
Metabolic
Trauma
Congenital
Vascular Stroke, arteriovenous malformation or fistula, cavernous angioma, granulomatous angiitis
Demyelination Multiple sclerosis
Neoplasm Epidermoid, dermoid, lipoma Hemangioblastoma Ependymoma Astrocytoma, ganglioglioma, xanthoastrocytoma, oligodendroglioma Leptomeningeal gliomatosis Intramedullary schwannoma Primary melanoma Metastasis Lymphoma
Inflammatory/infection AIDS, neurosyphilis, viral, vaccine, autoimmune Parasitic: cysticercosis, sparganosis, schistosomiasis, toxoplasmosis
Granuloma Sarcoid, tuberculosis, brucella, histoplasmosis, vasculitis
Vitamin deficiency Systemic illness, drug related

*Courtesy of Dr. Jack Rock, M.D.

well as immunoglobulin G (IgG) index, oligoclonal bands, and flow cytometry. The results were inconclusive. Steroids were given, and the patient eventually underwent rehabilitation. Repeat imaging was undertaken at a later time.

■ Discussion

Transverse myelitis is an inflammation of the spinal cord, which can occur in isolation or in the setting of another illness. It can occur after an infectious illness, postvaccinal, with systemic autoimmune diseases, from a vascular etiology, or as a prelude to multiple sclerosis. Lower extremity and bowel dysfunction is common.

The differential of a solitary intramedullary spinal cord lesion is extensive (**Table 36–1**). CSF should be sent to the laboratory for protein, glucose, cell count with differential, cytology, flow cytometry, oligoclonal bands, IgG index, immunology for B and T cells, Gram stain, aerobic and anaerobic cultures, as well as more esoteric cultures like viral, fungal, cryptococcal, lyme, and acid fast bacteria.

Because a spinal cord biopsy carries more risk than benefit, and will not likely change the treatment in these cases, it is usually not done. Steroids and rehabilitation are the mainstays of treatment. Usually improvement occurs in the first few weeks, but may take up to 2 years. One third of patients can return to almost normal function, one third recover but still have some deficit, and one third do not recover from the attack.

SUGGESTED READING

Krishnan C, Kaplin AI, Deshpande DM, Pardo CA, Kerr DA. Transverse myelitis: pathogenesis, diagnosis, and treatment. Front Biosci 2004;9:1483–1499

■ SECTION C ■

Lumbar

37

Discogenic Back Pain

■ Presentation

A 50-year-old man complained of low back pain and an L5 radiculopathy.

■ Radiologic Findings

Sagittal T2-weighted magnetic resonance imaging (MRI) of the lumbar spine is remarkable for a desiccated disc at L4–L5 (**Fig. 37–1**).

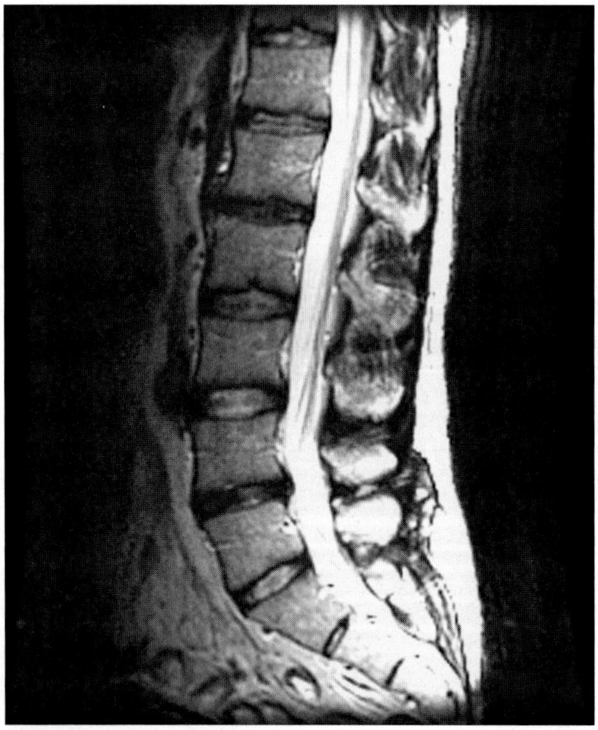

FIGURE 37–1 This T2-weighted sagittal lumbar MRI is remarkable for a desiccated L4–L5 disc.

■ Diagnosis

Degenerative disc

■ Treatment

A percutaneous single-level interbody and pedicle screw fusion was done.

■ Discussion

The annulus is the fibrous ring that surrounds the soft nucleus of the disc. The annulus is a ligament and can tear, producing back pain due to the pain fibers within its structure. This can be visualized on MRI, but is more definitively diagnosed on a provocative discography. On a discogram, the dye leaks out through a tear in the annulus.

The provocative discography can help identify the pain generator. It assesses four parameters: disc morphology, disc pressure, disc volume, and subjective pain. Provoking concordant pain in a patient with relevant history and a "good psychiatric profile" (in the presence of a negative control) has strong diagnostic value. One must realize there is interoperator variability to this test. Furthermore, overinjecting can provoke pain in even a normal disc. The presence of annular high signal intensity on an MRI has a high correlation with findings of an annular tear on discography; however, the latter has the ability to identify concordant pain.

Interbody fusions are becoming more widely accepted as a treatment option for discogenic back pain. Patients with such pathology typically present with mechanical low back pain with or without radiculopathy. They also have MRI findings of a single disc desiccation with decreased disc height or Modic II end-plate changes and a positive discography. Such patients usually benefit from fusion surgery.

Supplemental interbody fusion diminishes micromotion, boosts anterior column support, and restores disc and foraminal height. This helps to decompress the nerve root and provides a more physiologic lordosis, likely decreasing adjacent level stress.

SUGGESTED READING

Bono CM, Lee CK. Critical analysis of trends in fusion for degenerative disc disease over the past 20 years: influence of technique on fusion rate and clinical outcome. Spine 2004;29:455–463

38

Adjacent Segment Disease

■ Presentation

A 68-year-old woman with two previous fusions was diagnosed with a new L3 radiculopathy and quadriceps weakness.

■ Radiologic Findings

A preoperative lumbar x-ray shows retrolisthesis of L2 on L3 (**Fig. 38–1**). Preoperative myelogram shows an L2–L3 extradural block, secondary to disc herniation (**Fig. 38–2**). A postoperative lumbar x-ray shows the correction of the listhesis with extension of the decompression and fusion (**Fig. 38–3**).

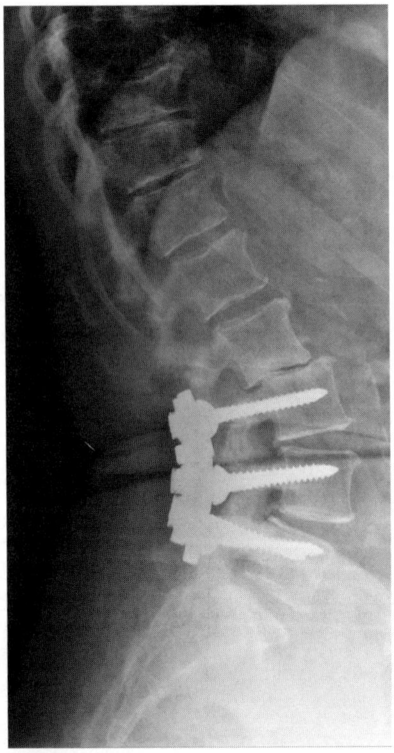

FIGURE 38–1 Preoperative lumbar x-ray with L2–L3 listhesis.

■ Diagnosis

Adjacent segment disease, with postfusion spondylolisthesis and disc herniation

■ Treatment

The patient's fusion and decompression were extended to incorporate the failed rostral level and the sacrum.

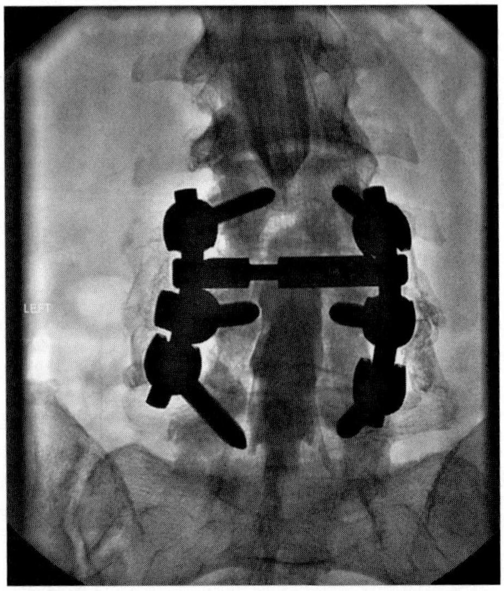

FIGURE 38–2 Myelogram demonstrating an epidural block.

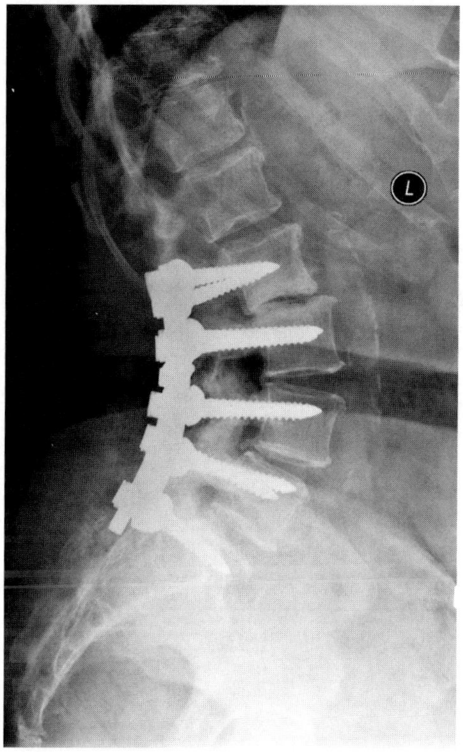

FIGURE 38–3 Postoperative x-ray with L2–S1 fusion and listhesis correction.

■ Discussion

Adjacent segment disease is a potential complication following fusion surgery. Debate has arisen as to whether this is the natural history of that segment in an already degenerative spine or whether this is iatrogenically accelerated. The answer is likely to be a combination of these processes. The differential of recurrent symptoms, or delayed symptoms after fusion surgery, is timeline related. In the days to weeks after surgery, infection will be a concern. In the first 3 to 6 months, pseudarthrosis with hardware failure is a possibility. Adjacent segment disease typically manifests itself in months to years after surgery.

The workup necessitates magnetic resonance imaging (MRI) with and without gadolinium, and possibly a computed tomography (CT) myelogram if there is too much metallic artifact to interpret the MRI. Dynamic spine x-rays, as well as blood work (sedimentation rate, CBC, cultures) and electromyography with nerve conduction velocities are also useful.

If a structural etiology is discovered, and further fusion surgery is planned, one must know the specifications of the already existing instrumentation. Knowing this preoperatively will enable the operating room staff to prepare the appropriate tools (screwdrivers, etc.) prior to the moment of utilization. The surgeon may plan to remove the existing instrumentation or link with it. Having the appropriate tools ready before beginning such an endeavor maximizes efficiency. When revising pedicle screws, one must be cognizant of thread type changes, as well as have other options of screw removal if the available drivers fail. Also important to revision fusion surgery is the ability to differentiate scar tissue from normal tissue. This is done by extending the incision to incorporate normal tissue planes rostrocaudally and using precaution when dissecting through scar tissue.

This patient had adjacent segment disease rostrally with instability. Her long-arm fusion had a "floating" rostral segment, and the new fusion was lengthened to accommodate it as well as the sacrum. While there is debate as to when S1 should be incorporated into a lumbar fusion, in the case of extant adjacent segment disease and multiple fused levels, the sacrum should be recruited into the construct for increased stability. Interbody fusion can help realign sagittal balance and reestablish disc height. However, if there is too much scarring, and the patient is elderly, the risks of this procedure may outweigh the benefits.

The recent introduction of motion sparing technology is meant to minimize adjacent segment disease. Its use is not applicable here due to the degree of three-column degenerative change, location, and other comorbidities. Nonetheless, the future development of this and other technology may change the incidence and the way adjacent segment disease is treated.

SUGGESTED READING

Javedan SP, Dickman CA. Cause of adjacent-segment disease after spinal fusion. Lancet 1999;354:530–531

39

Motion Preservation Technology

■ Presentation

A 39-year-old man had low back pain that was refractory to months of conservative therapy. The pain has altered his lifestyle.

■ Radiologic Findings

Lumbar magnetic resonance imaging (MRI) (sagittal T2-weighted) demonstrates an L4–L5 annular tear without other evidence of significant degenerative change (**Fig. 39–1**). Note the hyperintensity of the dorsal annulus.

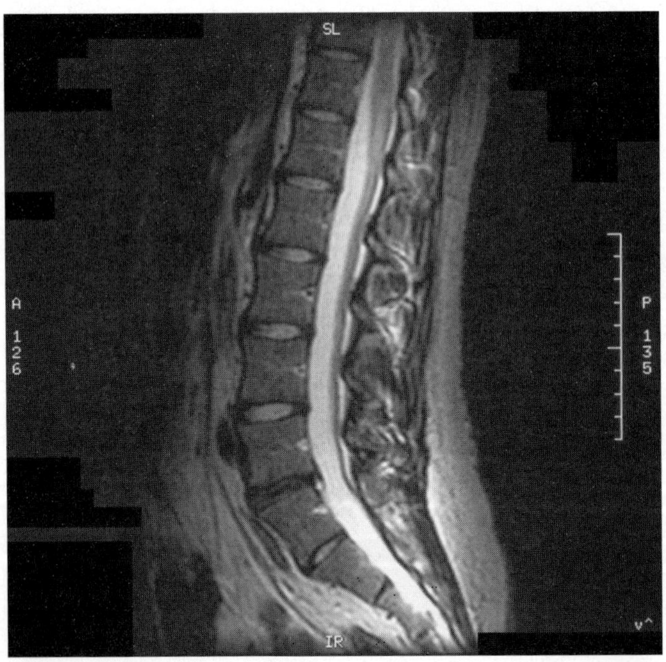

FIGURE 39–1 L4–L5 annular tear as seen on sagittal MRI of the lumbar spine.

■ Diagnosis

Annular tear

■ Treatment

This patient is a candidate for artificial disc implantation.

■ Discussion

Degenerative lumbar disc disease is prevalent in the middle-aged population. It is estimated that over 60 million Americans suffer lower back pain every year. Multiple treatments have been tried over the years for mechanical lower back pain secondary to degenerative disc disease (DDD). They range from facet rhizotomy, to indradiscal electrothermal therapy (IDET), and ultimately, to spinal fusion. It is estimated that about one quarter million people undergo fusion surgery every year in the United States alone.

Lumbar artificial discs have emerged as an alternative technique to relieve pain while preserving the motion segment. The artificial discs offer restoration of foraminal and disc heights and the reestablishment of normal lordotic curvature. These factors seem to contribute to a lesser occurrence of adjacent level disease sometimes seen with arthrodesis. The U.S. Food and Drug Administration has recently approved the Charité artificial disc (DePuy Spine, Raynham, Massachusetts). This is the first device for spinal disc replacement in the United States.

The Charité artificial disc is indicated for spinal arthroplasty in patients age 18 to 60 years, with adequate bone quality. Candidates should present with clinical and radiographic findings of single-level DDD between L4 and S1.

A 6-month trial of conservative therapy is needed prior to consideration for disc replacement surgery.

An MRI of the lumbar spine, flexion and extension lumbar x-rays, a full-length standing film to rule out scoliosis or other major spine deformity, and a dual energy x-ray absorptiometry (DEXA) scan are part of the preoperative workup. Contraindications are end-plate compromise (a vertebral body burst fracture or osteoporosis) or conditions that may compromise bone density (chronic anticonvulsant use, low estrogen levels). Surgery is not offered if the patient's bone mineral density is more than one standard deviation below the norm. Absolute contraindications are the presence of an uncontained disc herniation with or without radiculopathy, spinal canal or lateral recess stenosis, translational instability over 3 mm, spondylolysis, isthmic spondylolisthesis, and advanced facet disease or scoliosis.

The implantation utilizes a retroperitoneal approach, done in conjunction with a vascular or general surgeon and a spine surgeon. Patients with morbid obesity or multiple previous abdominal surgeries pose significant technical challenges and should be excluded. Pregnancy and infection are obvious contraindications as well.

In a prospective randomized study looking at neurologic complications and outcome following anterior lumbar interbody arthrodesis versus lumbar arthroplasty, the number of patients with major, minor, or other neurologic complications was equivalent. The Charité disc recipients had equivalent or better mean self-reported assessments when compared with the fusion patients.

SUGGESTED READINGS

Geisler FH, Blumenthal SL, Guyer RD, et al. Neurological complications of lumbar artificial disc replacement and comparison of clinical results with those related to lumbar arthrodesis in the literature: results of multicenter, prospective, randomized investigational device exemption study of Charité intervertebral disc. J Neurosurg Spine 2004;1:143–154

Griffith SL, Shelokov AP, Buttner-Janz K, LeMaire JP, Zeegers WS. A multicenter retrospective study of the clinical results of the LINK SB Charité intervertebral prosthesis. The initial European experience. Spine 1994;19:1842–1849

40

Percutaneous Lumbar Laminotomies and Foraminotomies

■ Presentation

A 48-year-old woman developed a left sciatic pain after a fall. She has failed months of conservative therapy. Neurologically, she has a positive straight leg raise in the left leg.

■ Radiologic Findings

There is mild spondylitic change with facet hypertrophy at L4–L5 and L5–S1, causing significant left foraminal stenosis at these levels. This is demonstrated on lumbar magnetic resonance imaging (MRI) (**Figs. 40–1** and **40–2**).

■ Diagnosis

Left L4 and L5 radiculopathy

■ Treatment

The patient received nerve conduction studies and also nerve root blocks. Her nerve conduction studies were positive for left L4 and L5 radiculopathies, and the nerve root blocks provided temporary relief. The patient was offered percutaneous left L4–L5, L5–S1 foraminotomies,

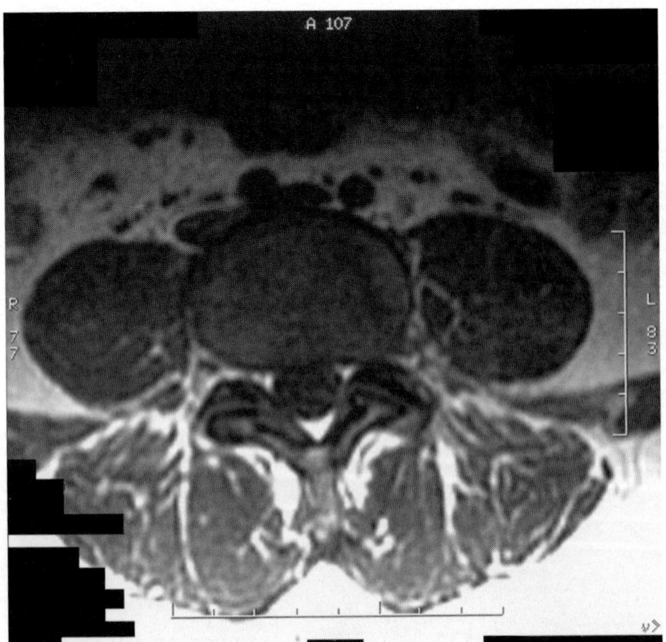

FIGURE 40–1 Axial MRI shows L4–L5 facet hypertrophy.

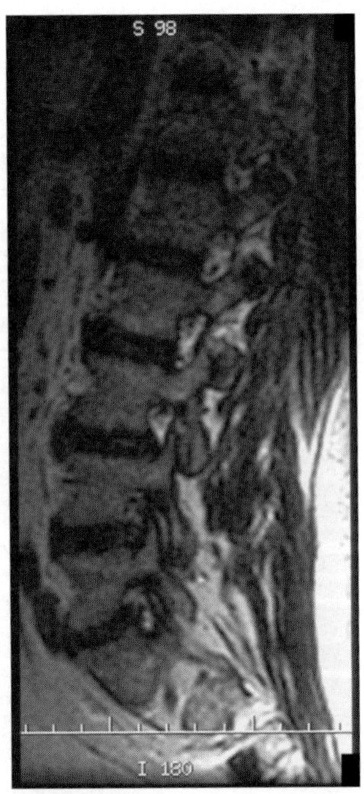

FIGURE 40–2 Sagittal MRI of the lumbar spine shows foraminal stenosis compressing the L4 and L5 exiting nerve roots.

and she agreed to surgery. Postoperatively, her symptoms improved.

■ Discussion

The recent refinement of percutaneous approaches has enhanced the surgical armamentarium of treatment options. Using any number of miniretractor systems, the surgeon can obtain direct access to the pathology with minimal blood loss and less disruption to the normal anatomy than traditional open techniques. This hastens recovery and improves patient outcomes. These surgeries are also offered in many centers as outpatient procedures.

SUGGESTED READING

Jenis LG, An HS, Gordin R. Foraminal stenosis of the lumbar spine: a review of 65 surgical cases. Am J Orthop 2001;30:205–211

41

Large Disc Herniation Treated Percutaneously

■ Presentation

A 46-year-old man had sudden-onset low back pain, with a right S1 radiculopathy that progressed over 2 months, despite physical therapy. He has mild dorsiflexion and extensor hallucis longus (EHL) weakness on the right.

■ Radiologic Findings

Magnetic resonance imaging (MRI) of the lumbar spine reveals a large disc extrusion, with sequestered fragment, occupying half the canal at the L5–S1 level (**Figs. 41–1** and **41–2**).

■ Diagnosis

Herniated lumbar disc

■ Treatment

A right L5–S1 microdiscectomy was completed.

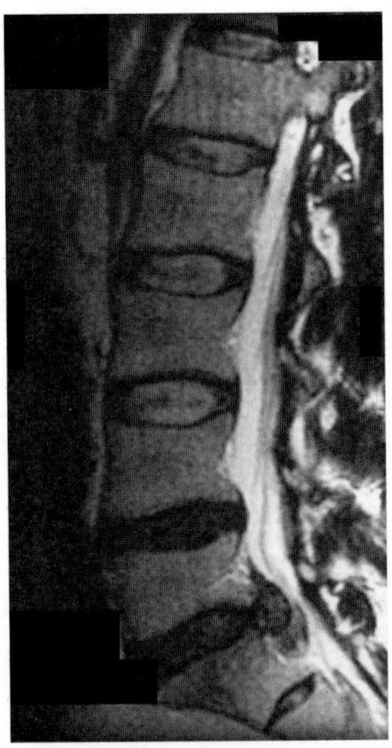

FIGURE 41–1 Sagittal MRI of the lumbar spine demonstrating disc herniation at L5–S1.

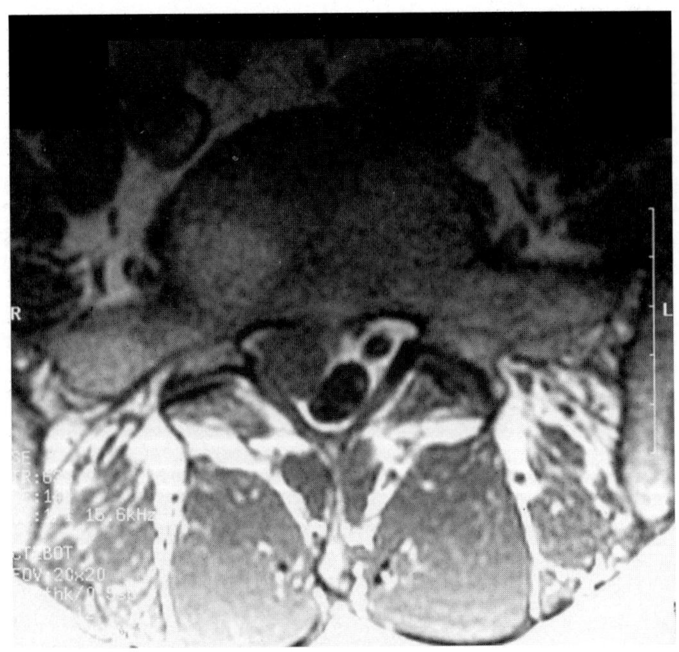

FIGURE 41–2 Axial MRI of the lumbar spine demonstrating disc herniation at L5–S1.

■ Discussion

Microdiscectomy has reached its final evolution as a technique. Using percutaneous minimally invasive technology, a small incision is created to minimize muscle trauma. Through this, large disc herniations, including calcified or sequestered fragments, can be removed in a timely manner with low morbidity. The patient recovered rapidly, and was able to return to work.

SUGGESTED READING

Nakagawa H, Kamimura M, Uchiyama S, Takahara K, Itsubo T, Miyasaka T. Microendoscopic discectomy (MED) for lumbar disc prolapse. J Clin Neurosci 2003;10:231–235

42

Segmental Instability

■ Presentation

A 37-year-old man presented with mechanical back pain after a previous discectomy. On examination, he had decreased sensation in the right L5 dermatome and limited lumbosacral flexion. Preoperative imaging demonstrated a mild disc bulge at L4–L5.

■ Radiologic Findings

Postoperative lumbar spine x-rays (**Figs. 42–1** and **42–2**) show interbody fusion and percutaneously placed pedicle screws at the L4 and L5 levels.

■ Diagnosis

Segmental instability

■ Treatment

The patient was treated with a percutaneous L4–L5 transforaminal lumbar interbody fusion and bilateral L4–L5 pedicle screw fixation and arthrodesis. At follow-up, he was pain free and able to return to work.

■ Discussion

Mechanical low back pain can sometimes become worse after a decompressive surgery. Segmental instability manifests as axial pain that is worsened by motion and improved by rest, which is typical of mechanical low back pain.

There is a differential for failed back syndrome, particularly in the immediate postsurgical period. Low back pain with fever and a reddened wound with discharge are obvious signs of infection. Persistence of a severe radiculopathy may represent a retained disc fragment, incorrect procedural level, or a complex regional pain syndrome. Magnetic resonance imaging (MRI) is an excellent diagnostic aid in these cases and should be done with and without gadolinium.

The differential expands in the weeks to months postoperatively. Recurrent radiculopathy may stem from perineural scar, another disc herniation, or adjacent level

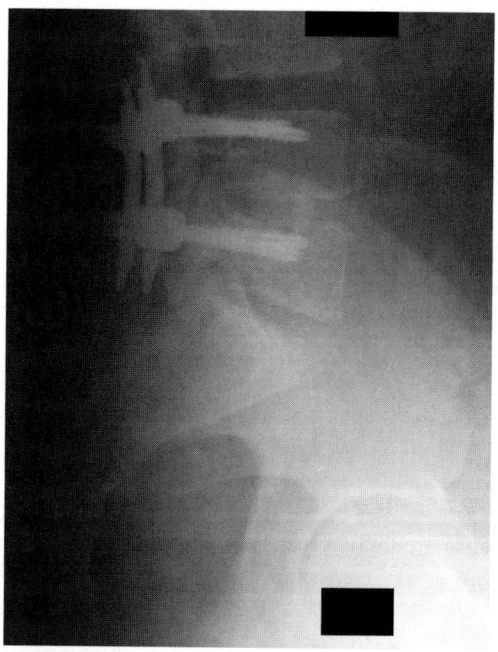

FIGURE 42–1 Lateral lumbar x-ray shows a single-level percutaneous fusion with pedicle screws and interbody fusion.

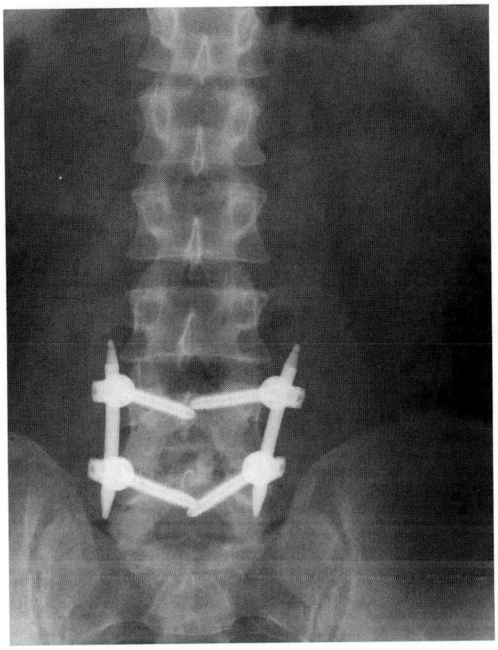

FIGURE 42–2 Anteroposterior lumbar x-ray shows a single-level percutaneous fusion with pedicle screws and interbody fusion.

herniation. Gradual development of mechanical back pain can represent segmental instability. Dynamic x-rays and facet injections can be employed as diagnostic tools for these cases. Fusion of the offending level eliminates the abnormal motion, which in turn provides satisfactory pain relief.

In this case, the patient's symptoms were mechanical, not radicular. There was little indication for further decompression, so a transforaminal lumbar approach provided a scar-free corridor to the disc space. Because this patient did not have a previous fusion, did not have scoliosis, and was not obese, he was a candidate for a percutaneous fusion. Interbody fusion offers a more physiologic reapproximation of sagittal balance and disc space height.

SUGGESTED READING

Kotilainen E. Long-term outcome of patients suffering from clinical instability after microsurgical treatment of lumbar disc herniation. Acta Neurochir (Wien) 1998;140:120–125

43

Lumbar Instability and Radiculopathy

■ Presentation

A 61-year-old woman with a history of rheumatoid arthritis who had four previous lumbar discectomies without fusion complains of chronic lumbar pain. She is neurologically intact. Magnetic resonance imaging (MRI) shows significant disc disease at L4–L5 and L5–S1 with decreased disc height and Modic end-plate changes.

■ Radiologic Findings

An axial highlight from the postmyelogram computed tomography (CT) reveals continued epidural compression on the right at the L5 level (**Fig. 43–1**).

■ Diagnosis

Recurrent degenerative disc disease

■ Treatment

This patient had a percutaneous two-level transforaminal lumbar interbody fusion (TLIF) and pedicle screw insertion (**Figs. 43–2** and **43–3**).

■ Discussion

Using a percutaneous pedicle screw insertion system (Sextant, Medtronic Sofamor Danek, Memphis, Tennessee), two-level lumbar fusions can be performed percutaneously through a minimal approach. Interbody fusions at L4–L5 and L5–S1 are done through small incision (Metrex tubular retractor, Medtronic Sofamor Danek). Through that same incision, pedicle screws can be inserted at L4 and S1 on that side, and through a small incision on the opposite side a similar procedure can be done. Postoperatively the patient went on to develop solid fusion and was pain free. Percutaneous pedicle screw insertion and fusion can provide an effective alternative to open fusion. In percutaneous cases, there is less muscle dissection and intraoperative blood loss, leading to better postoperative function and pain control. These techniques do have a steep learning curve, which must be overcome to optimize the results.

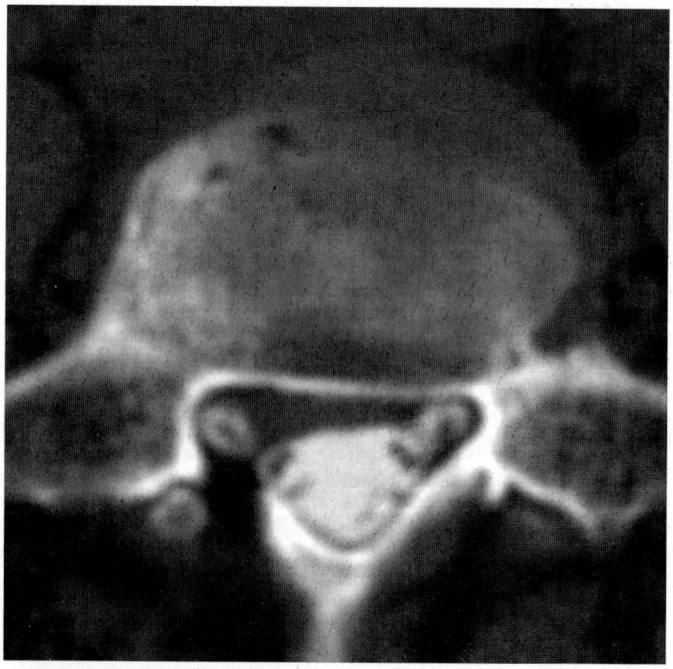

FIGURE 43–1 Postmyelogram CT demonstrates epidural compression.

▪ Discussion

Spondylolisthesis describes the anterior "slip" of one vertebral body over another. Grade I is 25% of anterolisthesis, grade II is more than 25 to 50%, grade III is more than 50 to 75%, and grade IV is a slip more than 75% the length of the vertebral body. Spondyloptosis is complete anterior translocation of one vertebral body in relation to the one below it.

Spondylolisthesis can be congenital, degenerative, or related to spondylolysis. Spondylolysis involves a defect between the superior articular process and the lamina. The superior articular process is attached to the body by the pedicle, but most of the lamina, inferior articular process, and spinous process is detached. This is most common at L5. It is typically seen as an elongated canal on axial imaging at the level of the defect. Patients are often asymptomatic, but symptoms can arise from instability or entrapment of the superior exiting nerve roots. These patients usually progress to surgery for decompression and fusion.

Multiple surgical techniques have been described to treat this lesion, and usually involve a posterior approach to the spine. The specifics of surgery ultimately depend on the symptoms, severity of listhesis, and its cause. While reduction can provide a mechanically sound construct, especially if interbody fusion is done, there is risk of further entrapping the exiting nerve roots. This risk is higher if reduction is attempted without axial distraction and prior to performing a wide facetectomy.

SUGGESTED READING

Beutler WJ, Fredrickson BE, Murtland A, Sweeney CA, Grant WD, Baker D. The natural history of spondylolysis and spondylolisthesis: 45 year follow-up evaluation. Spine 2003;28:1027–1035

46

High-Grade Spondylolisthesis

■ Presentation

A 52-year-old woman complained of chronic mechanical low back pain radiating to the thighs. On examination, sensation was decreased in the L5 distribution bilaterally. She had limited lumbosacral extension, with some paraspinous muscle spasm, and negative straight leg raises. Also, she had grade II spondylolisthesis at L5–S1 on lumbar x-ray.

■ Radiologic Findings

A postoperative x-ray demonstrates transpedicular screws and rods at L4, L5, and S1, with a T-piece fusion mass (**Fig. 46–1**).

■ Diagnosis

High-grade spondylolisthesis

■ Treatment

A 270-degree fusion, with L4–S1 decompression, pedicle screw fixation, and arthrodesis was performed.

■ Discussion

Spondylolisthesis is most common at the L5–S1 level and may come from several causes, including congenital, traumatic, pathologic, degenerative, or isthmic. Isthmic spondylolisthesis is also known as spondylolysis and is due to a pars fracture. Spondylolisthesis has four grades: I (less than 25% subluxation), II (25% to 50% subluxation), III (greater than 50% to 75% subluxation), and IV (greater than 75% subluxation). These patients present with mechanical low back pain and often some form of radiculopathy stemming from significant foraminal compromise as well as disc derangements at the slipped level. When there is evidence of radiculopathy or claudication or severe mechanical low back pain, decompression and fusion are the preferred procedures; otherwise, conservative management may be employed. To work toward eliminating micromotion, interbody fusion can be used

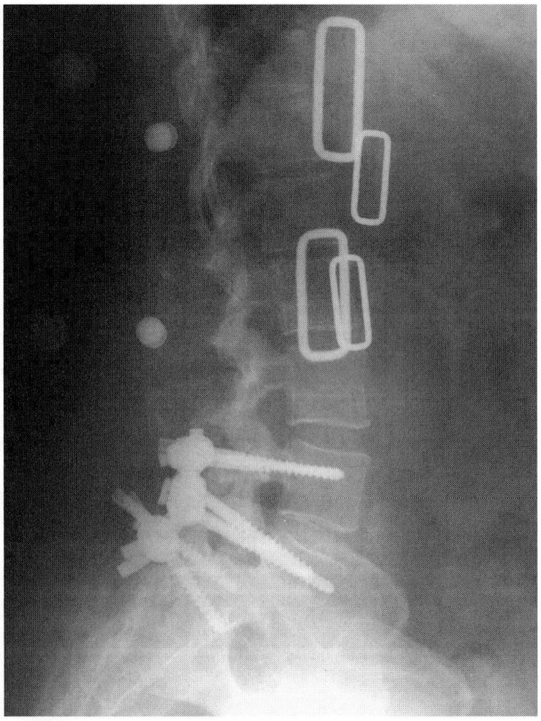

FIGURE 46–1 Postoperative lumbar x-ray with transpedicular screws and rods are noted at L4, L5, and S1, with a T-piece fusion mass.

to augment this construct, leading to a 270-degree fusion from one entry point. In some cases, an anterior-posterior approach may be necessary to achieve mechanical stability and solid fusion.

SUGGESTED READING

Bozkus H, Dickman CA. Transvertebral interbody cage and pedicle screw fixation for high-grade spondylolisthesis. Case report. J Neurosurg 2004;100:62–65

47

Multilevel Posterior Lumbar Interbody Fusion

■ Presentation

A 44-year-old woman presented with chronic mechanical low back pain and antalgic weakness of the hip flexors. She has an obese habitus and is a heavy smoker.

■ Radiologic Findings

T1-weighted magnetic resonance imaging (MRI) of the lumbar spine shows degenerative changes at L3–L4 and L4–L5, with decreased disc space height, anterior osteophytes, and Modic end-plate changes indicating anterior column instability. There is multilevel lumbar facet hypertrophy as well (**Fig. 47–1**).

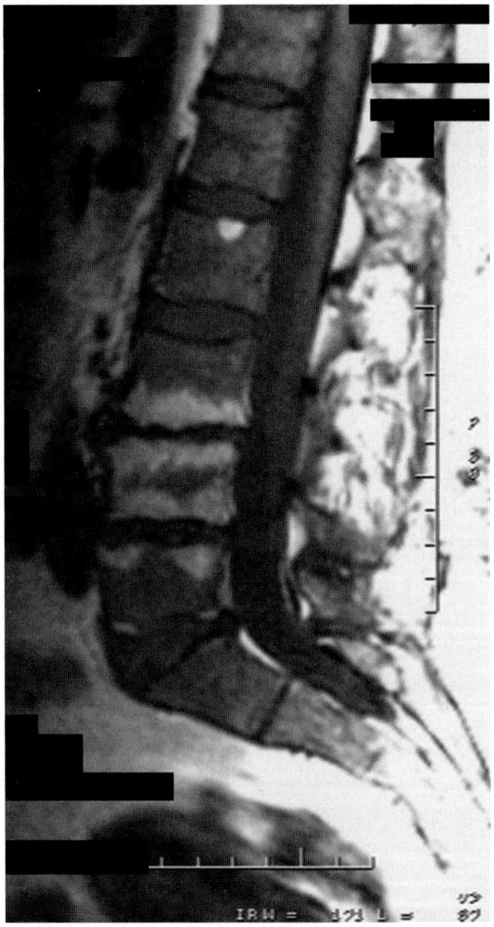

FIGURE 47–1 MRI of the lumbar spine shows multilevel degenerative changes, including Modic type II changes at L3–L4 and L4–L5.

■ Diagnosis

Lumbar instability

■ Treatment

This patient had bilateral L3–L4, L4–L5 laminectomies and posterior lumbar interbody fusions, with an L3–S1 pedicle screw fixation.

■ Discussion

The presence of Modic end-plate changes indicates anterior column instability, which typically presents with severe mechanical back pain. Following interbody fusion, with more normal restoration of disc height, mechanical back pain improves significantly when compared with posterolateral fusion alone.

Modic end-plate changes are classified into three types. Type I changes show increased signal intensity on T2-weighted sequences. Type II changes shows high intensity on T1- and T2-weighted sequences. If the bone sclerosis is extensive, but the signal intensities are decreased on T1- and T2-weighted sequences, this is a type III change.

This patient has several risk factors for nonunion: obese habitus, nicotine habit, multiple levels of fusion, and the redo nature of this case. The definition of "fusion" is occasionally an area of debate. Fusion can be defined by two criteria: clinical and radiographic. Clinically, the resolution of mechanical low back pain postoperatively is a criterion. Radiographic fusion denotes the finding of a solid, uninterrupted bony fusion mass across the fused segments with the absence of a bone/graft interface on x-ray. In the case of structural allograft, this may take months. Additionally, lack of movement across the fused segment on flexion/extension x-ray and no signs of graft resorption or halo signs around the screws is part of the definition. To help improve this patient's fusion rate, she is maintained in an external orthosis and received a bone stimulator.

SUGGESTED READINGS

Couture DE, Branch CL Jr. Posterior lumbar interbody fusion with bioabsorbable spacers and local autograft in a series of 27 patients. Neurosurg Focus 2004;16:E8

Modic MT, Masaryk TJ, Ross JS, Carter JR. Imaging of degenerative disk disease. Radiology 1988;168:177–186

48

Bone Morphogenetic Protein

■ Presentation

A 48-year-old woman presents with mechanical low back pain and a history of an L3–S1 pedicle screw fusion as well as L4–L5, L5–S1 interbody fusion. Dynamic films show instability across L4–L5 and L5–S1, indicating the development of nonunion.

■ Radiologic Findings

As seen on axial computed tomography (CT) myelogram, there are soft tissue filling defects, likely due to postoperative fibrosis, at L4–L5 and L5–S1. Transverse process bony formation was minimal (**Fig. 48–1**).

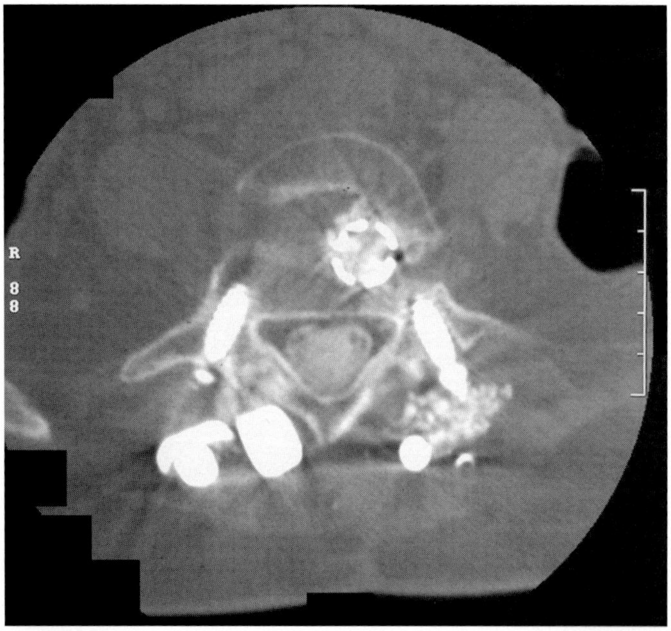

FIGURE 48–1 CT myelogram demonstrating an incomplete fusion mass.

■ Diagnosis

Lumbar instability

■ Treatment

Redo lumbar spinal fusion with bone morphogenetic protein.

■ Discussion

This patient had numerous risk factors for nonunion, including nicotine use, nonuse of external orthosis after the initial surgery, and a history of pelvic radiation. She needed a revision surgical fusion, and was an excellent candidate for bone morphogenetic protein to enhance her fusion chances. Recent advances in osteoinductive substances have caused a resurgence of interest in determining which technique offers a more reliable, faster, solid fusion. Specifically, bone morphogenetic protein (Medtronic Sofamor Danek, Memphis, Tennessee) has been approved by the U.S. Food and Drug Administration (FDA) for use in anterior spinal fusion, but has been used off label elsewhere according to surgeon discretion. Its proponents boast that bone morphogenetic protein has a better fusion rate than allograft or autograft for all patients, including smokers. Graft substitution offers a great alternative to iliac crest harvest, which carries some morbidity, such as harvest site pain, bleeding, and infection. These morbidities can be eliminated by graft substitution. However, the high cost of this new technology can be a drawback.

SUGGESTED READING

Burkus JK, Heim SE, Gornet MF, Zdeblick TA. The effectiveness of rhBMP-2 in replacing autograft: an integrated analysis of three human spine studies. Orthopedics 2004;27:723–728

49

Degenerative Scoliosis

■ Presentation

A 59-year-old woman complains of mechanical back pain with radiculopathy that has been ongoing for a year, despite nonsurgical treatment. On examination she had antalgic weakness of the right hip flexors and extensors and limited lumbosacral flexion.

■ Radiologic Findings

Magnetic resonance imaging (MRI) (T2-weighted sagittal, **Fig. 49–1**) showed degenerative scoliosis from L1 to S1 with degenerative disc disease. Postoperative lumbar x-ray (**Fig. 49–2**) reveals T12–S1 pedicle screw fixation with cross-linkage.

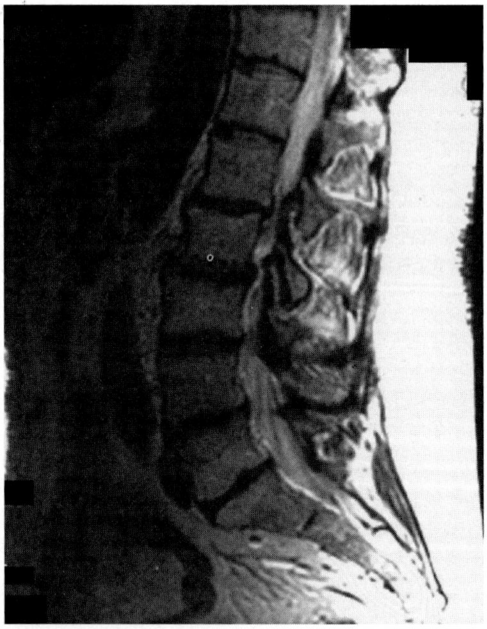

FIGURE 49–1 MRI of the lumbar spine shows a scoliotic spine with spondylostenosis.

■ Diagnosis

Degenerative scoliosis

■ Treatment

A multilevel decompression and T12 to S1 pedicle screw fixation using iliac crest graft and a bone stimulator were completed. The patient's preoperative pain resolved.

■ Discussion

Mechanical back pain has many etiologies, including scoliosis. Degenerative scoliosis is the end result of advanced degenerative spine disease. As wear and tear increases on the discs, excessive motion ear stress a preexisting deformity. It is not uncommon for people to present with unilateral multilevel radiculopathies secondary to the biomechanics of the concavity.

Treatment options for degenerative scoliosis depend on the patient's symptoms. Mechanical lower back pain, the presence of neurologic symptoms or radiculopathy, the type of curve, and the overall clinical condition are factors to consider. If the main presentation is that of radiculopathy, decompression alone or with a short segmental fusion may suffice in an elderly patient with focal instability and suboptimal health status. On the other hand, in a younger, healthier patient presenting with significant mechanical low back pain and instability (a lateral, anterior, or rotational listhesis), a reconstructive multilevel segmental fusion is a good option. Either way,

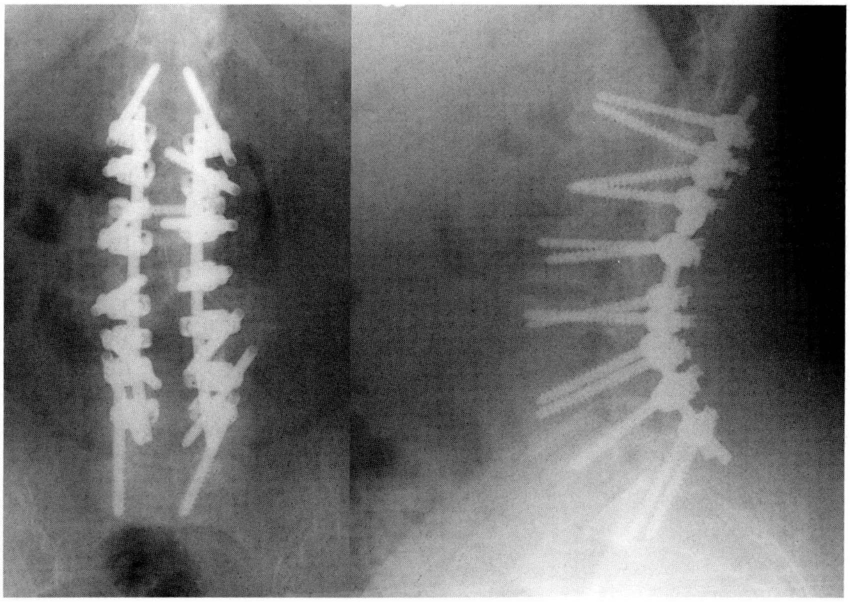

FIGURE 49–2 AP and lateral x-rays of the postoperative construct display a T12 to S1 pedicle screw fusion.

assessment of sagittal balance will drive the treatment plan.

A posterior approach alone is appropriate in a milder, less rigid curve and when severe canal stenosis is encountered. An anteroposterior (AP) approach has the advantages of restoring anatomic balance and disc and foraminal height, and achieves a superior fusion rate. This combined approach is recommended in stiff, less reducible curves with somewhat more osteopenic bone quality.

A dramatic increase in surgical risk is encountered in patients over 60 years of age. For this population, the nutritional status pre- and postfusion should be optimized. Beware of the use of any anticoagulation (Coumadin, heparin, Lovenox, etc.), and encourage early mobilization. Intraoperative monitoring as well as the intraoperative wake-up test are valuable resources. Special attention to the caudal aspect of arthrodesis is necessary, as there is a pattern of failure relating to the lower part of the fusion.

SUGGESTED READING

Gupta MC. Degenerative scoliosis. Options for surgical management. Orthop Clin North Am 2003;34:269–279

50

Nerve Root Impingement by Pedicle Screw

■ Presentation

A 52-year-old woman presented with significant mechanical low back pain, sciatica, and extensor hallucis longus weakness. Her straight leg raise was positive on the left, and she had limited lumbosacral flexion. In the immediate postoperative setting after a percutaneous fusion, she reported radicular pain.

■ Radiologic Findings

Preoperatively, computed tomography (CT) myelogram showed L4–L5 grade I spondylolisthesis and a small disc herniation at that level. Postoperatively, CT myelogram demonstrated a broad lateral extradural impression from the L4–L5 to the L5–S1 disc space level. Impingement of the pedicle screw on the exiting root was noted (**Fig. 50–1**).

■ Diagnosis

- Lumbar instability
- Pedicle screw misplacement with nerve root impingement

■ Treatment

Initially, the patient had a percutaneous left L4–L5 discectomy, transforaminal lumbar interbody fusion (TLIF), and pedicle screw fixation. After developing a radiculopathy, she underwent an open procedure, involving removal of lumbar instrumentation, replacement of bilateral L4–L5 pedicle screws, morselized bone graft arthrodesis, and transverse lumbar interbody fusion. She achieved a good recovery after the second surgery.

■ Discussion

Percutaneous pedicle screw fixation is a newer technology with tissue preservation advantages, less blood loss, and better functional outcomes. However, the learning

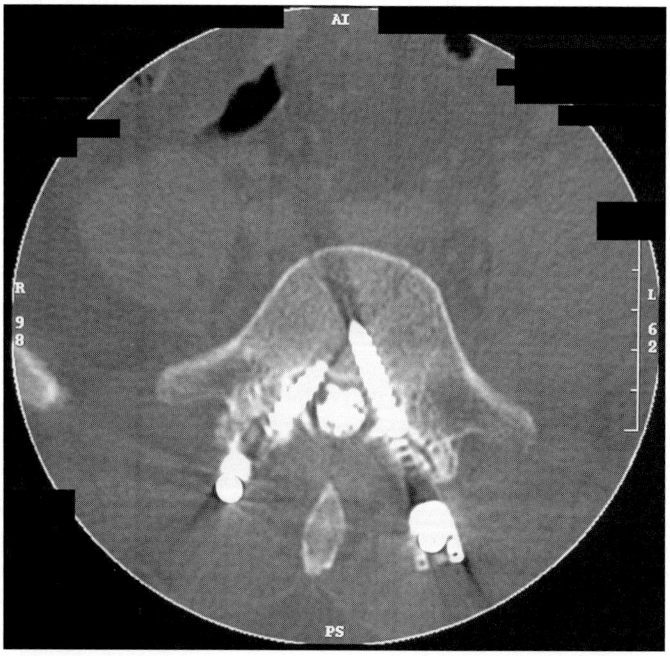

FIGURE 50–1 CT myelogram with pedicle screws impinging on nerve roots.

curve is steep, and there is limited visualization of the anatomy in comparison with open techniques. Dependence on intraoperative fluoroscopy or image navigation is essential, as well as an innate understanding of the anatomy. Intraoperative electromyography and serial postoperative examinations are also instrumental for patient safety in these cases.

This patient had an early percutaneous fusion, and as the technique increased in use, complications lessened. Again, the postoperative examination is important, as well as early imaging, if the symptoms indicate it. Nerve root impingement symptoms can improve if caught early.

SUGGESTED READING

Wiesner L, Kothe R, Schulitz KP, Ruther W. Clinical evaluation and computed tomography scan analysis of screw tracts after percutaneous insertion of pedicle screws in the lumbar spine. Spine 2000;25:615–621

51

Lumbar Scoliosis

■ Presentation

A 58-year-old man complained of progressive mechanical low back pain, radiating down his right lower extremity. He has antalgic weakness of the proximal lower extremities and decreased lumbar flexion. Magnetic resonance imaging (MRI) of his lumbar spine demonstrated degenerative scoliosis with multilevel stenosis with spondylolisthesis.

■ Radiologic Findings

Anteroposterior (AP) x-ray of the lumbar spine shows an L1–S1 rod and screw construct with a bone stimulator (**Fig. 51–1**).

■ Diagnosis

Degenerative scoliosis

■ Treatment

An L1–L5 decompression was completed with L1–S1 bilateral pedicle screw fusion with arthrodesis and reduction of scoliosis.

■ Discussion

Scoliosis has been classified into two types: structural or nonstructural (postural, inflammatory, compensatory, etc.). The latest classification by the Scoliosis Research Society includes idiopathic, neuromuscular, congenital, neurofibromatosis, mesenchymal, rheumatoid, traumatic, osteochondral dystrophies, infectious, metabolic, degenerative, or tumorous types of scoliosis.

Adult scoliosis is a type of deformity that has its onset in adulthood, secondary to progressive multilevel disc degeneration leading to asymmetric loss of disc height along with facet degeneration and osteopenia. This contributes to progressive deformity of the spinal segment,

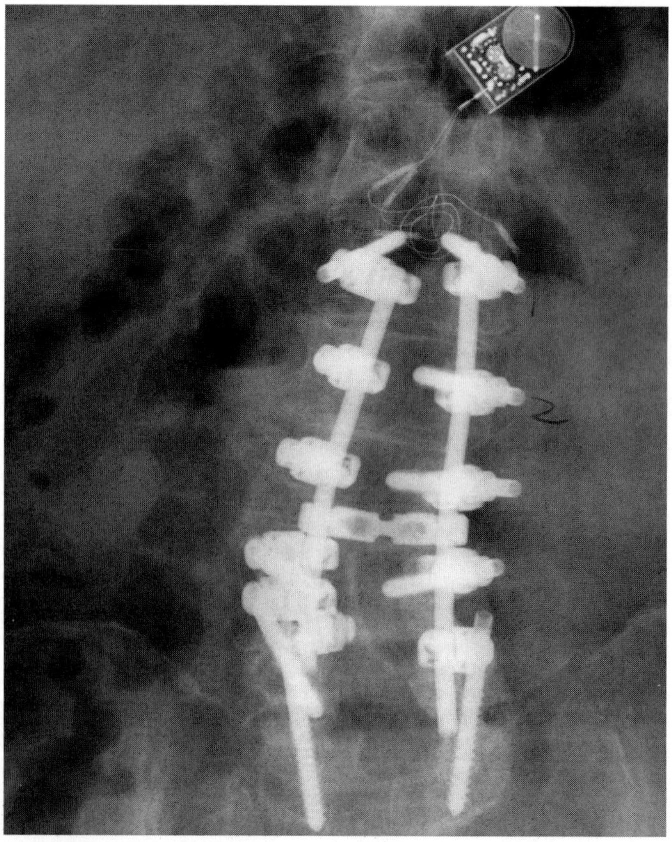

FIGURE 51–1 AP lumbar x-ray showing an L1 to S1 pedicle screw fusion with a bone stimulator.

which can be measured with Cobb angles. The typical presentation is that of spinal stenosis and asymmetric radiculopathies secondary to foraminal stenosis. Axial pain is more frequent on the convex side due to muscle fatigue, and the radicular pain usually stems from the concave side.

The workup consists of radiographic evaluation, comparison with older films, and ruling out other systemic pathology. Nonsurgical treatment focusing on postural correction can be attempted, but adult deformity is usually rigid, and these issues are determined on a case-by-case basis. Surgery is indicated to decompress the neural elements or to correct a painful deformity.

A relatively flexible thoracic curve or a balanced double major curve can respond well to posterior fixation. On the other hand, rigid or unbalanced curves usually require additional anterior releases. A common complication with long arm fusion is the development of nonunion manifesting as hardware failure. A good arthrodesis technique with careful bone preparation, the use of a bone stimulator, and the addition of graft substitutes such as bone morphogenetic protein (BMP) are helpful pearls for avoiding pseudarthrosis. It is important to note that BMP has not yet been approved for this type of use.

SUGGESTED READING

Tribus CB. Degenerative lumbar scoliosis: evaluation and management. J Am Acad Orthop Surg 2003;11:174–183

52

Degenerative Lumbar Spine Disease with Segmental Instability

■ Presentation

A 62-year-old woman presented with pain on lumbar flexion but was otherwise intact. Dynamic lumbar films demonstrated a mobile listhesis at L3–L4. She has had two lumbar laminectomies and has a chronic history of mechanical low back pain.

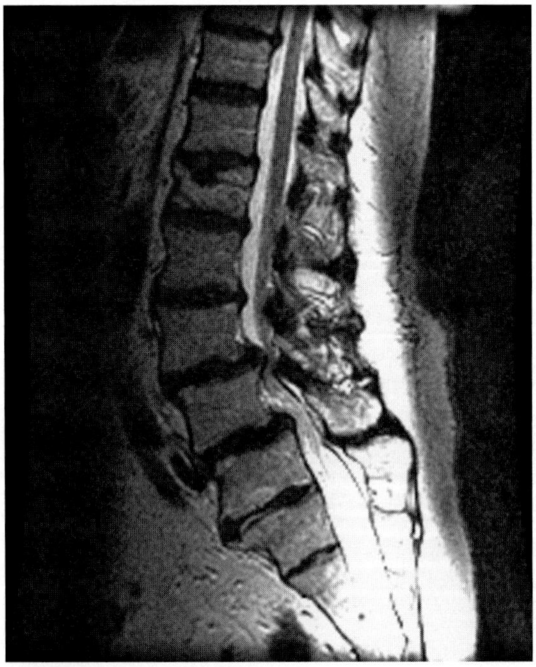

FIGURE 52–1 Sagittal lumbar MRI demonstrating multiple levels of degenerative discs with associated posterior element changes.

■ Radiologic Findings

T2-weighted magnetic resonance imaging (MRI) of the lumbar spine shows severe spondylotic change throughout, with Modic end-plate changes at L3–L4, L4–L5, and L5–S1 (**Fig. 52–1**).

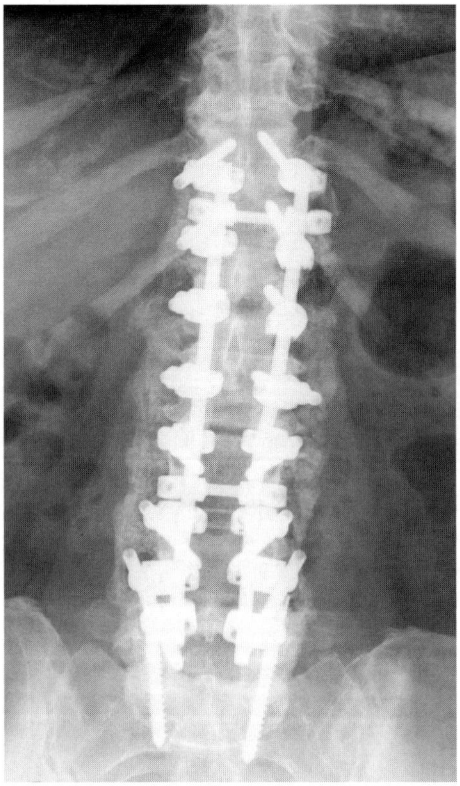

FIGURE 52–2 T11–S1 pedicle screw fusion with cross-links and T-piece fusion.

■ Diagnosis

Multilevel spondylitic changes with instability

■ Treatment

A T11–S1 pedicle screw fusion was performed and is viewed on anteroposterior (AP) x-ray (**Fig. 52–2**).

■ Discussion

This patient has failed previous conservative treatment. Although one could perform a pedicle screw fixation at L3–L4, this would not address her entire pathology and would put additional stress on the other degenerated levels. The optimum treatment in this case is a multilevel segmental fusion from T11–S1, which incorporates her pain generators and instability, and does not stress the thoracolumbar junction. Postoperative follow-up demonstrated a fusion mass and an improvement in her symptoms.

SUGGESTED READING

Braithwaite I, White J, Saifuddin A, Renton P, Taylor BA. Vertebral end-plate (Modic) changes on the lumbar spine MRI: correlation with pain reproduction at lumbar discography. Eur Spine J 1998;7:363–368

53

Lumbar Nonunion

■ Presentation

A 45-year-old man underwent an L5–S1 fusion for grade II spondylolisthesis 4 years ago and in recent months has started suffering a progressive mechanical low back pain. He is neurologically intact.

■ Radiologic Findings

Flexion/extension lumbar x-rays show mobile, grade II spondylolisthesis, with poor bony formation and a fractured S1 screw (**Fig. 53–1**).

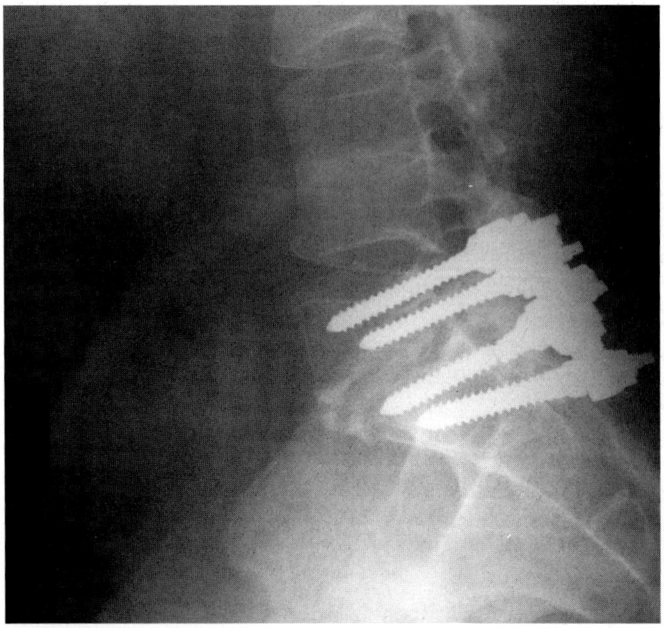

FIGURE 53–1 Previous lumbar fusion with nonunion and a fractured S1 screw.

■ Diagnosis

Pseudarthrosis

■ Treatment

The patient had an L5–S1 anterior interbody fusion with femoral ring allograft.

■ Discussion

Nonunion is a risk of any fusion surgery. Risks for developing nonunion include smoking, morbid obesity, previous surgery, multilevel fusion, metabolic disorders such as diabetes mellitus, osteoporosis, and certain medications such as nonsteroidal anti-inflammatory drugs (NSAIDs) or steroids. Nonunion is a surgical problem and can be treated in a variety of ways.

Anterior lumbar interbody fusion (ALIF) is preferred in a patient with previous posterior fusion who presents with nonunion (mechanical low back pain) but without radiculopathy or other signs of neural element compression. Otherwise a redo posterior fusion will be necessary. Rarely do we resort to combined 360-degree fusion. Highlighted risks of ALIF are retrograde ejaculation and urethral or vascular injury.

This patient underwent an anterior lumbar interbody fusion and achieved a solid union. The recent introduction of osteoinductive materials such as bone morphogenetic protein has enhanced fusion rates, making nonunion less frequent.

SUGGESTED READING

Lee C, Dorcil J, Radomisli TE. Nonunion of the spine: a review. Clin Orthop 2004;419:71–75

54

Mechanical Back Pain with Previous Posterior Fusion

■ Presentation

A 45-year-old man who had a previous L5–S1 fusion continued to have mechanical back pain a few months postoperatively. Workup demonstrated nonunion. He is without neurologic deficit.

■ Radiologic Findings

Five months after his initial posterior surgery, the graft failed to be incorporated (**Fig. 54–1**). This indicates nonunion.

■ Diagnosis

Nonunion

■ Treatment

An anterior lumbar interbody fusion (ALIF) was done (**Fig. 54–2**). The patient's previous cage was removed and then replaced with bilateral cages containing bone morphogenetic protein (BMP).

■ Discussion

The question of whether to fuse a patient from the front or the back has been a source of debate. If the pathology is posterior (a migrated disc fragment, facet hypertrophy, lateral recess stenosis), the recommended approach is posterior. This approach is also preferred if the patient has had abdominal surgery, has severe atherosclerosis, or is a male of reproductive age. If the patient has already had a posterior surgery, an anterior approach is preferred to avoid scarring, augment a fusion, or address vertebral body pathology.

In this case, we weighed the options of redo posterior fusion, ALIF, or a pain procedure (such as morphine pump). Because the patient had a previous posterior approach, anterior fusion was chosen. A pain procedure

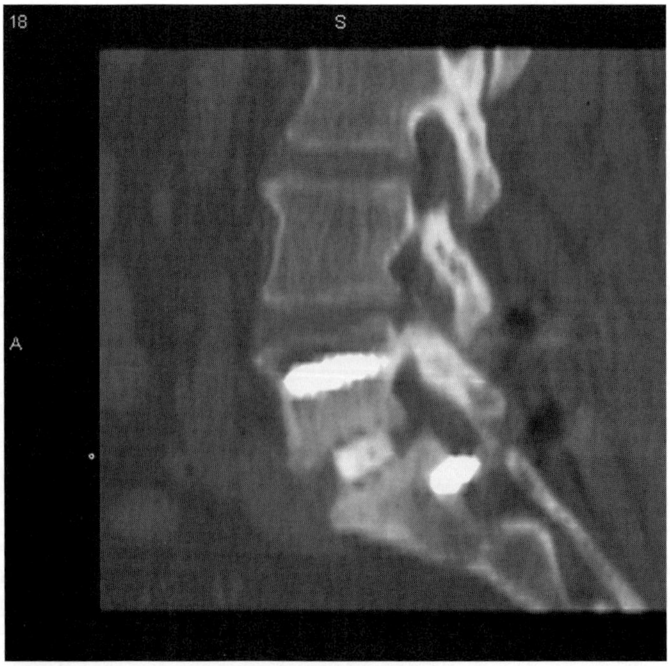

FIGURE 54–1 Computed tomography (CT) reconstruction of the lumbar spine demonstrates pseudarthrosis of his previous fusion attempt.

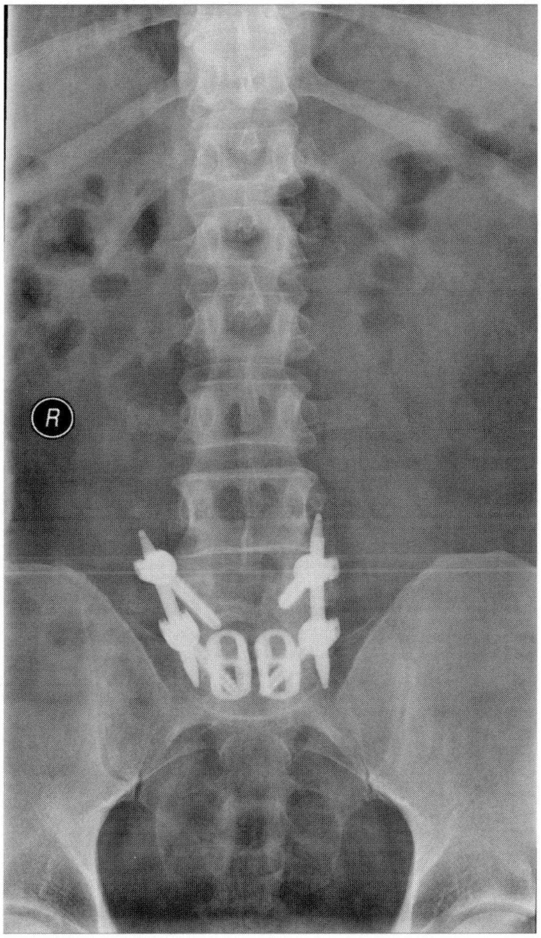

FIGURE 54–2 Postoperative construct as seen on anteroposterior (AP) lumbar x-ray.

could be considered if there wasn't a structural pathology that could be improved safely through surgery. In this case, an ALIF with BMP in a cage was performed with success.

SUGGESTED READING

Duggal N, Mendiondo I, Pares HR, et al. Anterior lumbar interbody fusion for treatment of failed back surgery syndrome: an outcome analysis. Neurosurgery 2004;54:636–643

55

Osteoporosis

■ Presentation

An 81-year-old woman fell from a standing position and developed intractable low back pain with radiculopathy. She was neurologically intact, but her pain increased with standing and walking. Her workup revealed focal lumbar stenosis with L1 and L4 osteoporotic compression fractures.

■ Radiologic Findings

Magnetic resonance imaging (MRI) of the lumbar spine demonstrated lumbar stenosis with L1 and L4 compression fractures (**Fig. 55–1**).

■ Diagnosis

Osteoporosis with spinal stenosis and compression fractures

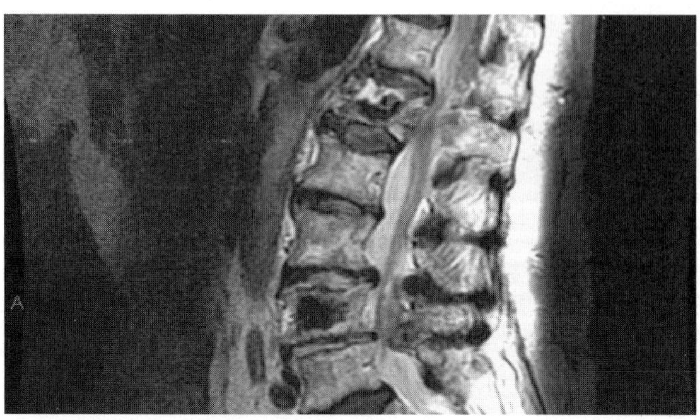

FIGURE 55–1 Sagittal T2-weighted MRI shows significant degenerative stenosis with associated compression fractures.

■ Treatment

The patient underwent percutaneous L1, L4, and L5 decompressions, followed by L1 and L4 kyphoplasties. The kyphoplasties were done in the operating room after the decompression, through a transpedicular route. The result can be seen in **Fig. 55–2**.

■ Discussion

Osteoporosis is a prevalent disease in which the cortical bone becomes too porous. It is estimated that over 50% of Caucasian women experience an osteoporotic fracture in their lifetime. In 2003 there were 1.5 million osteoporotic fractures in the United States alone, 50% of which involved the vertebral bodies and 25% involved the hip.

The typical patient is an elderly Caucasian woman with a small habitus and positive family history. The use of certain

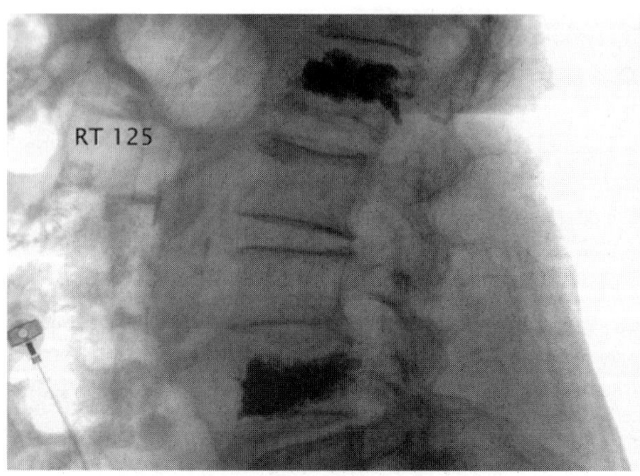

FIGURE 55–2 Lateral fluoroscopic image demonstrates the completion of the L1 and L4 kyphoplasties.

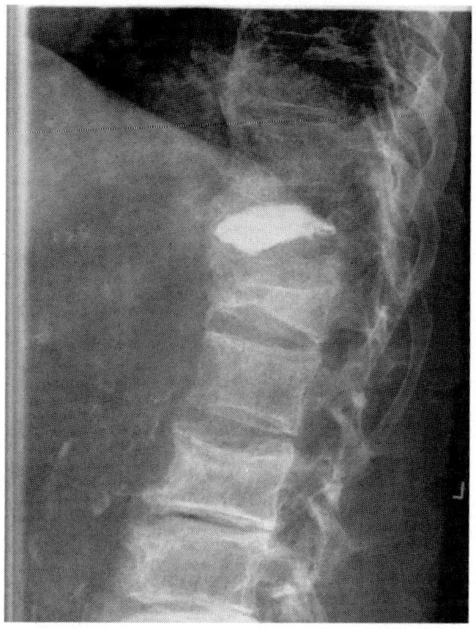

FIGURE 55–3 One can see the results of a T12 kyphoplasty, and also an L1 compression fracture.

medications, such as steroids, and some chemotherapy can accelerate osteoporosis. In addition, alcohol and tobacco use coupled with inadequate calcium intake can augment the severity of this bone loss.

The incidence of fractures from seemingly nontraumatic events increases exponentially in the eighth decade for women who have low bone density. While prevention, nutrition/exercise, and pharmaceutical treatment are the mainstay, surgical intervention also has a role.

The treatment of an osteoporotic compression fracture has three key factors: (1) overall assessment of bone quality, (2) addressing the compression fracture, and (3) pharmaceuticals. The underlying pathology must be treated. A bone densitometry should be performed on all postmenopausal women with risk factors as well as women presenting with osteoporotic compression fractures. In addition, a bone and mineral specialist can help coordinate pharmaceuticals—calcium and vitamin D supplementation and the use of calcium "fusing" agents—and address lifestyle changes and how to decrease other risk factors.

The compression factor itself has to be addressed. An acutely painful fracture is a surgical indication. Acute fractures have increased signal on T2 in the vertebral body from marrow edema, as well as active intake on bone scan. An MRI with gadolinium is needed to rule out other reasons for the fracture (i.e., neoplasm) and evaluate for neural compression. Chronic or painless fractures are not surgical indications, unless there is progressive kyphosis. If neural compression is the surgical indication, decompression can be done. Fusion hardware failure is a real risk in this group because of bone quality, previous medications, and age.

Kyphoplasty has been successful in treating the painful compression fractures of osteoporosis. This procedure, usually done percutaneously, involves restoring vertebral body height and alignment by inflating a balloon, and then securing the correction by filling the space with bone cement. Patients report pain reduction and higher activity tolerance. This can also be an outpatient procedure.

Vertebroplasty is less expensive but has a higher rate of cement extravasation due to the high-pressure injection. Furthermore, it does not reduce the fracture or restore normal spine mechanics. Prophylactic treatment is a source of debate but makes biomechanical sense, at least at the thoracolumbar junction.

Both kyphoplasty and vertebroplasty have potential complications, usually related to the effects of cement extravasation or access issues. The results of a T12 kyphoplasty and also an L1 compression fracture are demonstrated on x-ray (**Fig. 55–3**). The L1 fracture developed months after the kyphoplasty. The question is whether the fracture is procedure related or disease-process related. The methylmethacrylate has a greater density than osteoporotic bone, and this may stress an already compromised level. In addition, the natural history of osteoporosis dictates additional fracture development. Although the clinical course can give some idea as to the etiology, adjacent level disease should be monitored. Because this new fracture was not painful, no invasive treatment was done.

How these procedures relieve pain is debatable. Pain relief is thought to result from stabilization of the fractured vertebrae. Reduction of postural kyphosis (more so following kyphoplasty) seems to further enhance the mechanics of the spine, decrease delayed deformity, and improve pain. It is speculated that the exothermic reaction generated by methylmethacrylate injection causes denervation of the periosteal nerve endings. This seems to contribute to pain control. Furthermore, thermal injury by methylmethacrylate is cytotoxic to tumor cells when used for contained spine metastases.

Percutaneous bone augmentation techniques cannot be offered in cases of traumatic fractures unrelated to osteoporosis, or in the presence of a three-column injury, or when retropulsion with neurologic compromise is identified. The presence of a vertebral body arteriovenous malformation can pose a bleeding risk when performing this procedure. Similarly, the presence of an old "scarred-down" fracture or severe scoliosis can create technical difficulty.

SUGGESTED READINGS

Phillips FM, Ho E, Campbell-Hupp M, McNally T, Wetzel F, Gupta P. Early radiographic and clinical results of balloon kyphoplasty for the treatment of osteoporotic vertebral compression fractures. Spine 2003;28:2260–2265

Ryu KS, Park CK, Kim MC, Kang JK. Dose-dependent epidural leakage of polymethylmethacrylate after percutaneous vertebroplasty in patients with osteoporotic vertebral compression fractures. J Neurosurg 2002;96:56–61

■ PART IV ■

Neoplasm

56

Metastatic Lesion

■ Presentation

An 85-year-old man with a history of prostate cancer complained of middle back pain, refractory to pain management. He had a thoracic sensory level, mild weakness of his lower extremities, and no other systemic signs of illness.

■ Radiologic Findings

Magnetic resonance imaging (MRI) of the thoracic spine shows a circumferential compressive lesion at T9 (**Figs. 56–1** and **56–2**).

■ Diagnosis

Metastatic lesion to the spine

■ Treatment

A transfacet-transpedicular approach was undertaken for decompression, followed by a long arm instrumented fusion (**Fig. 56–3**).

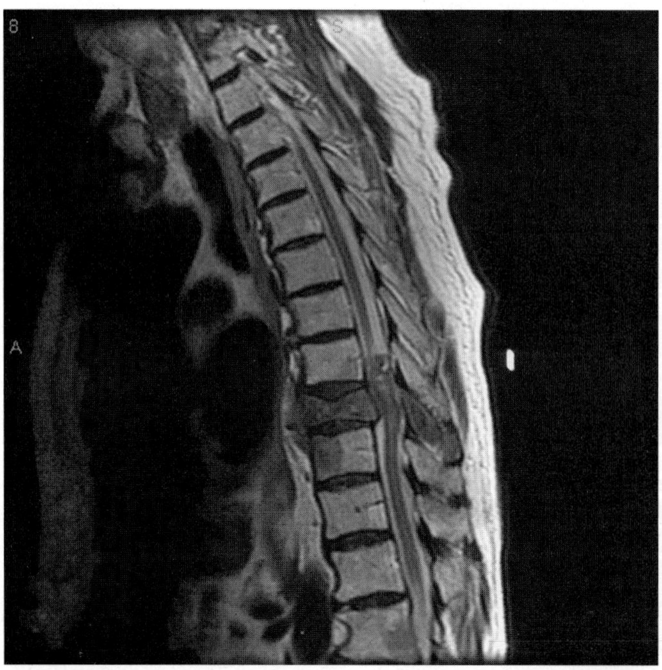

FIGURE 56–1 Sagittal MRI of the thoracic spine demonstrates a thoracic bony lesion.

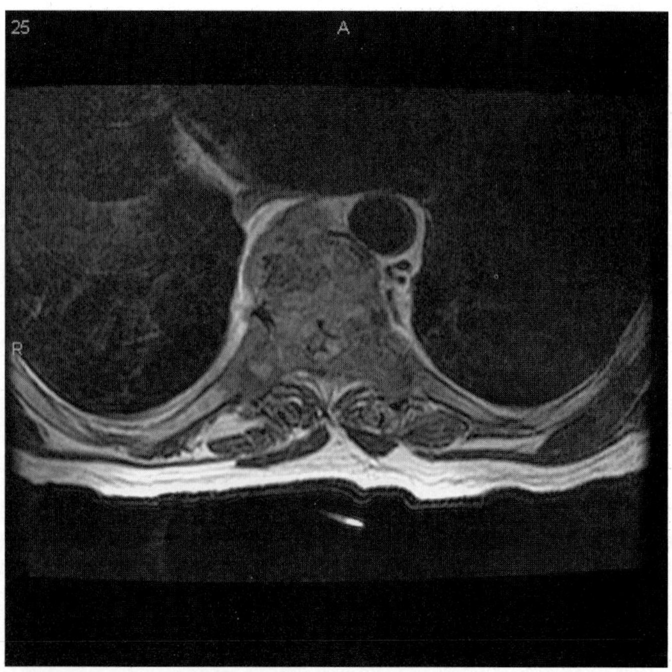

FIGURE 56–2 Axial MRI of the thoracic spine demonstrates the circumferential nature of metastatic lesions to the spine, which can allow a transpedicular approach.

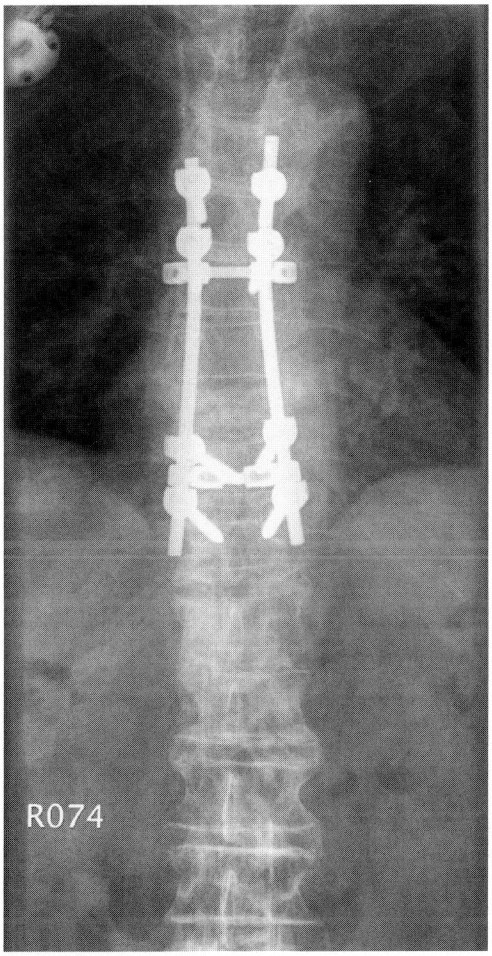

FIGURE 56–3 Thoracic anteroposterior (AP) x-ray with thoracic pedicle screw fusion.

■ Discussion

Metastatic lesions to the spine are usually spread through a hematogenous route, with lung, breast, gastrointestinal tract, and prostate being the most common primary sources. The thoracic spine is the most common location, followed by the lumbar spine, and over half of the patients with metastatic lesions have multiple lesions. Usually the bony column is affected, but epidural spread can be seen. About 10% of patients with cancer present with metastatic spine lesions at the initial assessment.

In the case of a patient who has a single compressive metastatic lesion, an acute incomplete neurologic deficit, and more than 3 to 6 months of life expectancy, and who can medically tolerate surgery, decompression and fusion is warranted. A transfacet, transpedicular approach affords direct access to the tumor. The destructive nature of these lesions allows an easy resection through the tumor-infested facet, pedicle, and even into the vertebral body through one approach.

Our institution has an institutional review board (IRB)–approved protocol for stereotactic radiosurgery to spine metastases. If a patient has one to three focal vertebral metastases with minimal neurologic deficit or pain, he or she gets radiation to the 90% line to cover the entire target. For a patient who has the same number (one to three) of lesions, but significant or rapidly progressive neurologic deficit, surgery is the first option. If the patient has diffuse vertebral metastases, but less than three are symptomatic, radiosurgery is offered for the symptomatic ones. Patients with diffuse symptomatic metastases get external beam radiation with possible additional radiosurgery.

SUGGESTED READINGS

Gerrard GE, Franks KN. Overview of the diagnosis and management of brain, spine, and meningeal metastases. J Neurol Neurosurg Psychiatry 2004;75(Suppl 2):37–42

Rock J, Ryu S, Yin F, Rosenblum M, Kim JH. A technique for intensity-modulated spinal radiosurgery. Presented at the Advanced Techniques in Image-Guided Brain and Spine Surgery meeting, New York, December 2003

57

Plasmacytoma with Postembolization Swelling

■ Presentation

A 52-year-old man with new-onset atraumatic back pain was found to have a large T6–T7 vertebral body lesion causing significant cord compression. Following preoperative embolization, he developed progressive right lower extremity weakness.

■ Radiologic Findings

Axial magnetic resonance imaging (MRI) of the thoracic spine reveals a right T6 and T7 paraspinal mass involving the vertebral bodies with cord compression (**Fig. 57–1**). Angiogram with T6 and T7 intercostal injections showed a neovascular stain and a hypervascular mass (**Fig. 57–2**).

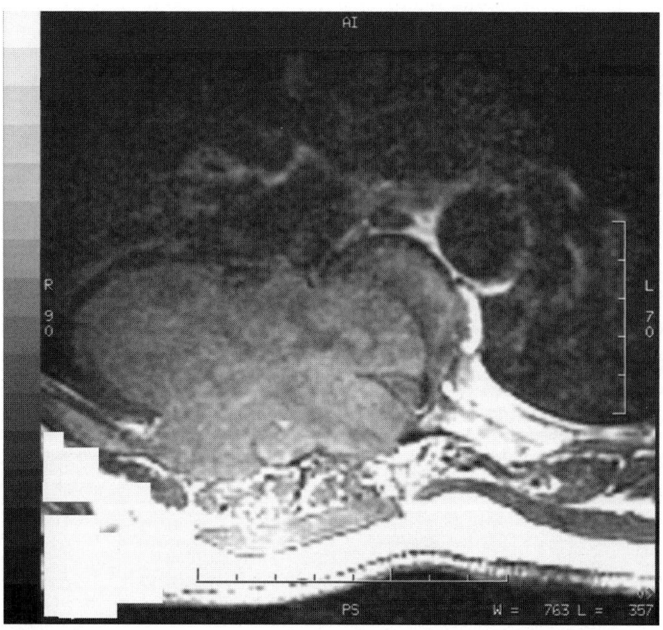

FIGURE 57–1 MRI with a compressive paraspinal mass.

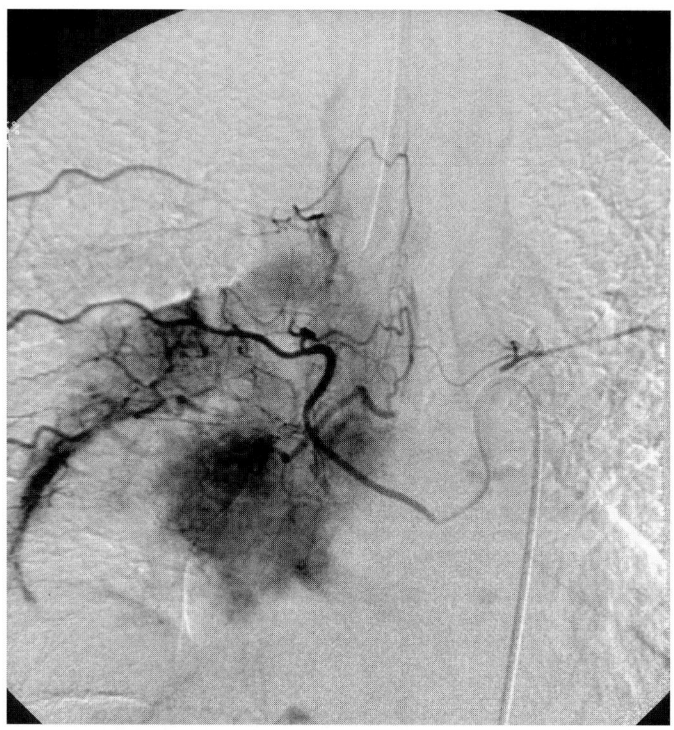

FIGURE 57–2 Angiogram demonstrating injection of a hypervascular mass.

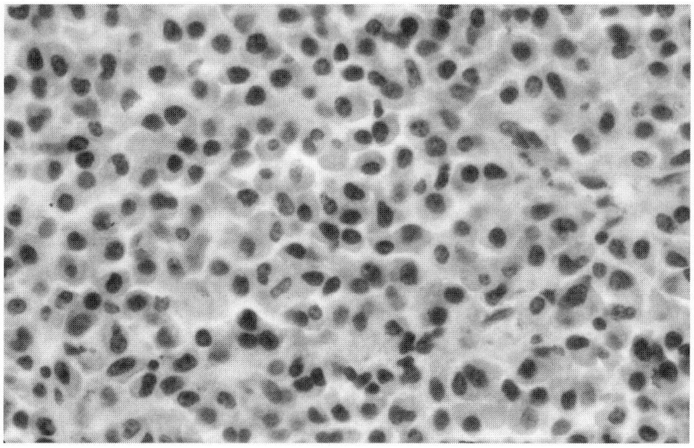

FIGURE 57–3 Histopathology slide of plasmacytoma.

■ Diagnosis

This patient had a plasmacytoma; atypical plasma cells are exhibited in a histopathology specimen (**Fig. 57–3**).

■ Treatment

This patient had an emergent right lateral extracavitary approach for T6 and T7 corpectomies with a T5–T8 fibular strut allograft and T3–T10 fusion and arthrodesis (**Fig. 57–4**). Postoperatively, he had stereotactic radiosurgery (14 Gy) to the spine. At follow-up, he had made an excellent recovery, was ambulatory, and was able to return to work.

■ Discussion

Plasmacytoma commonly presents as a solitary thoracic lesion with signs of cord compression. It is a radiosensitive tumor, but with the significant amount of cord compression found in this case, there was concern that radiosurgery could have further compromised the cord. Moreover, the size of this tumor made the radiosurgical option less attractive.

Preoperative embolization, in an effort to minimize blood loss during surgery, is advisable because these tumors are quite vascular. Postembolization, 1 to 2% of patients can experience difficulties, such as parent vessel occlusion, cord infarct, acute tumor necrosis, and swelling with further neurologic deficit. The latter can occur following radiation treatment also. The treatment then is to give steroids and perform emergent surgery.

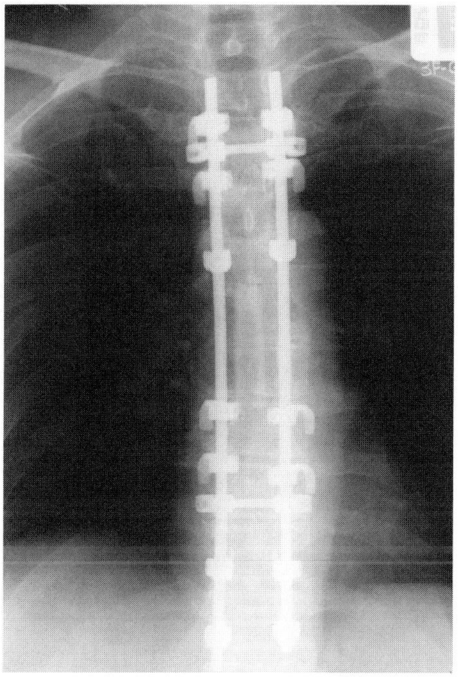

FIGURE 57–4 Postoperative x-ray with the construct displayed.

The extracavitary approach is a useful way for the surgeon to operate on all three columns through one approach. Access to intra- and extraspinal elements is available, and is ideal for addressing anterolateral and dorsal compression from tumor, trauma, or infection in association with kyphotic deformity. Although this is a major surgery, it negates the need for a thoracotomy, and thus is called the "one-and-a-half" approach.

SUGGESTED READING

Takahashi T, Koshu K, Tominaga T, Takahashi A, Yoshimoto T. Solitary plasmacytoma in the thoracic spine. Two case reports. Neurosurg Rev 1998;21:121–125

58

Thoracic Tumor

■ Presentation

A 57-year-old woman had long-standing thoracic pain. She had brisk reflexes, but no other neurologic signs. An extensive medical workup was significant for a mass extending from the spinal canal, through the foramen, and under her sixth rib.

■ Radiologic Findings

T2-weighted magnetic resonance imaging (MRI) demonstrated a hyperintense soft tissue mass displacing the thoracic cord and extending through the neural foramen (**Figs. 58–1** and **58–2**).

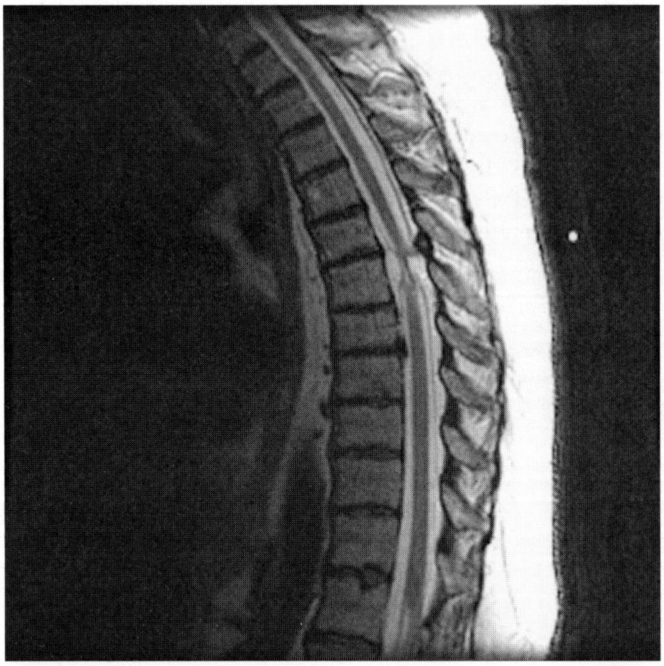

FIGURE 58–1 Sagittal MRI of the thoracic spine reveals a soft tissue mass displacing the cord.

■ Diagnosis

The pathologic specimen, a mixture of adipose and vessels, was an angiolipoma

■ Treatment

A T6 lateral extracavitary approach was performed for lesion excision.

■ Discussion

Although the typical spinal intraforaminal lesions are schwannomas, neurofibromas, and sometimes

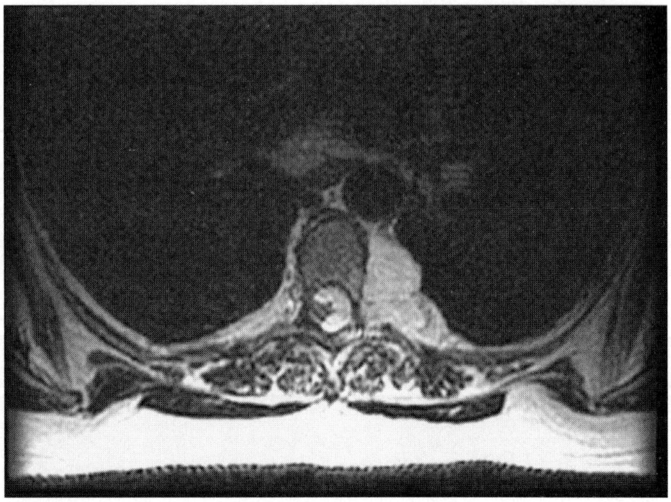

FIGURE 58–2 Axial MRI of the thoracic spine again shows the cord displacement and foraminal extension.

meningiomas, rarer lesions should be considered in the differential. An angiolipoma is a rare benign fatty tumor composed of mature lipocytes and multiple areas of angiomatous elements. It can be noninfiltrating, located in the subcutaneous tissue, or infiltrating, found in the deep soft tissue. It is benign and can be cured by surgical excision.

The lateral extracavitary approach is a good option for patients with thoracic intraspinal tumors that have an extraforaminal/intrathoracic extension. This approach lets the surgeon decompress the canal and follow the residual tumor to the chest cavity all in one approach. This technique is contraindicated in elderly patients with severe cardiopulmonary compromise; the duration of this surgery and the amount of blood loss and fluid exchange can have higher morbidity.

SUGGESTED READING

Fourney DR, Tong KA, Macaulay RJ, Griebel RW. Spinal angiolipoma. Can J Neurol Sci 2001;28:82–88

59

Thoracolumbar Instrumentation Failure

■ Presentation

A 70-year-old woman presented with metastatic breast cancer and cord compression. She had previously undergone decompression and fusion for acute cord compression. Postoperatively, she regained some ambulation, then presented 3 weeks later with acute back pain and wound dehiscence.

■ Radiologic Findings

The upper thoracic construct failed, as demonstrated on the lateral thoracic x-ray (**Fig. 59–1**).

■ Diagnosis

Hardware extrusion

■ Treatment

The patient underwent a wound irrigation and debridement with revision of her thoracolumbar fusion.

■ Discussion

Patients with metastatic spine disease are a challenge when major surgery is planned. The decision making is multifactorial. Life expectancy, the compromised quality of pathologic bone, staging, and overall condition are considered. Additionally, the degree of spine involvement, the presence or absence of cord compression, neurologic status, bone quality, and the patient's outlook on the disease and a possible major surgery must all be contemplated.

If the decision to go to surgery has been made, the option of anterior versus posterior approach is weighed.

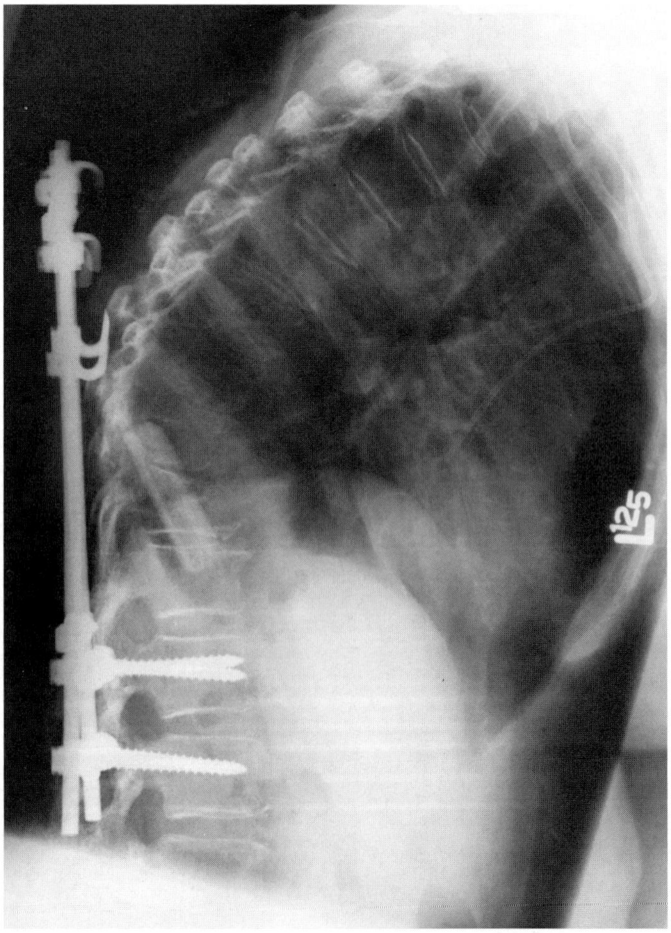

FIGURE 59–1 Thoracic x-ray demonstrating hardware pullout superiorly.

Deciding factors include the degree of vertebral involvement and primary location of compression in the sagittal and coronal planes. Posterior segmental fusion provides a solid fixation with rods and hooks and/or pedicle screws. Structuring an opposing claw configuration helps provide secure fixation points at each end of the construct, if hooks and claws are used. Three-dimensional correction can be delivered through a single dorsal approach.

Severe osteoporosis, active infection, or the absence of adequate ventral column support can make the construct more failure prone. On the other hand, attention to the anatomy, meticulous bony preparation for arthrodesis, adequate and healthy graft, an external orthosis, and perhaps the addition of a bone stimulator can make failure a less likely event. In addition, one may consider a plastic surgery consult in regard to flap planning and prevention of hardware extrusion.

SUGGESTED READING

Manstein ME, Manstein CH, Manstein G. Paraspinous muscle flaps. Ann Plast Surg 1998;40:458–462

60

Thoracic Screw Misplacement

■ Presentation

A 53-year-old man with known metastatic lung cancer to the spine complained of pleuritic chest pain following a transpedicular approach for a T7 corpectomy and T5–T9 pedicle screw fixation and arthrodesis.

■ Radiologic Findings

Computed tomography (CT) of the thoracic spine shows pedicle screw misplacement (**Fig. 60–1**).

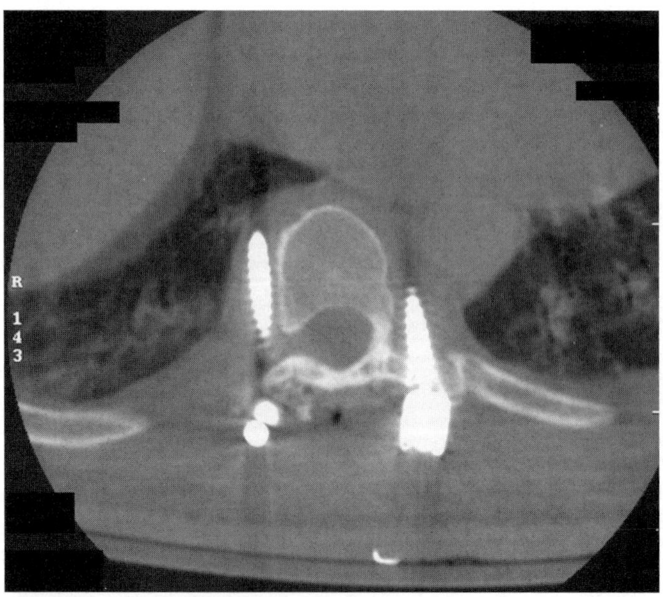

FIGURE 60–1 Axial CT of the thoracic spine shows misdirected thoracic pedicle screws.

■ Diagnosis

Extrapedicular screw placement

■ Treatment

The patient underwent revision surgery.

■ Discussion

When compared with a hook and rod construct, posterior thoracic fixation using pedicle screws provides instant three-column rigid fixation using a relatively short construct. This construct allows unloading of the incompetent ventral elements in patients too sick to undergo ventral or 360-degree surgery. Pedicle screws are also valuable in delayed kyphosis cases when the lamina has already been removed, obviating the use of hook or sublaminar wires. Thoracic pedicle cannulation is contraindicated in pathologically compromised or anatomically unfit ("almond-shaped") pedicles.

Variability exists among spine surgeons as to the best trajectory for pedicle cannulation. Knowing the level, shape, and size of the pedicle, its coronal and sagittal relationship to the rest of the spine, as well as the surrounding anatomy is prerequisite for performing a safe pedicle screw placement. CT imaging and careful preoperative planning is essential. Intraoperative image guidance or fluoroscopy may further enhance pedicle screw placement.

SUGGESTED READING

Belmont PJ Jr, Klemme WR, Dhawan A, Polly DW Jr. In vivo accuracy of thoracic pedicle screws. Spine 2001;26:2340–2346

61

Recurrent Giant Cell Tumor

■ Presentation

A 29-year-old man initially presented with low back pain and bilateral radiculopathies. He had a posterior resection of an S1 lesion followed by 48 Gy external beam radiation. A few months later, he had recurrent bilateral S1 radiculopathies without bowel, bladder, or sexual dysfunction. On examination, he had decreased sensation in the left S1–S3 dermatomes, absent left ankle jerk, and left plantar flexion weakness.

■ Radiologic Findings

On magnetic resonance imaging (MRI) of the lumbosacral spine, there is a bony destructive lesion involving the left S1 segment, extending into the canal. It displaces the thecal sac and impinges on the S1 nerve root (**Figs. 61–1** and **61–2**).

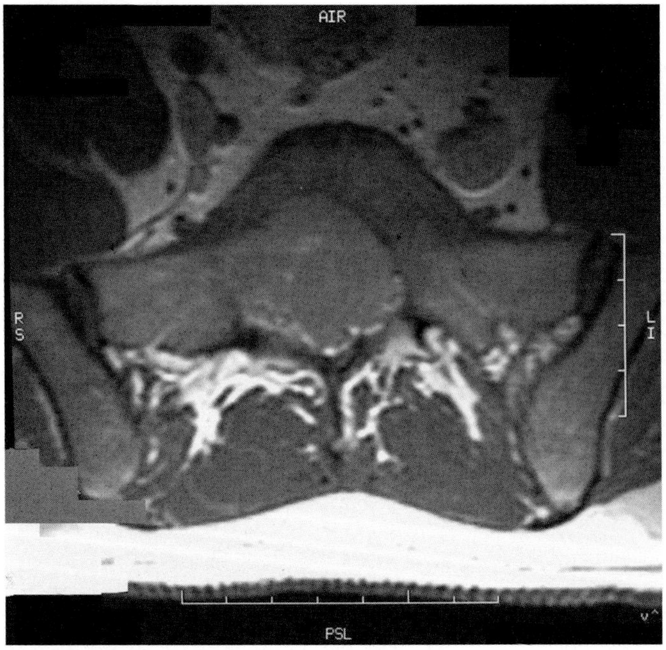

FIGURE 61–1 Axial MRI scan showing a destructive sacral lesion impinging on the canal.

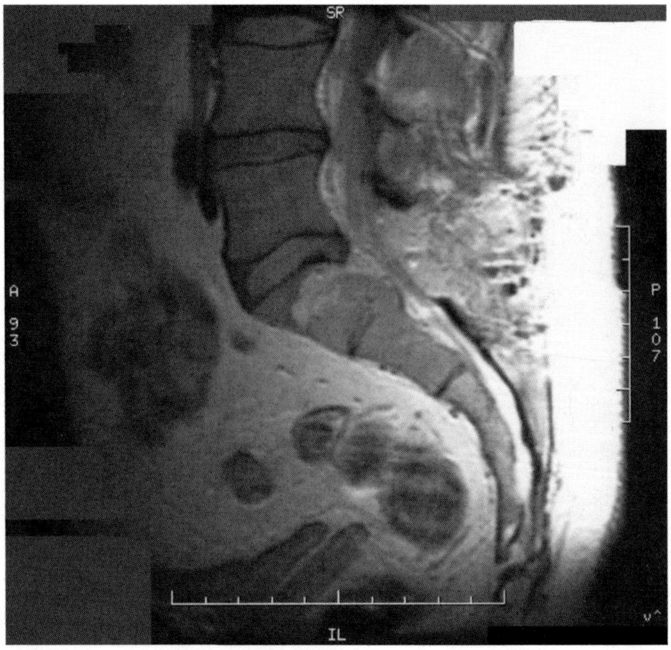

FIGURE 61–2 Sagittal MRI displays a lesion, destroying bone and extending into the spinal canal.

64

Benign Thoracic Tumor

▪ Presentation

A 55-year-old woman had a year and a half of history of midthoracic pain with a sensory deficit and bowel and bladder dysfunction. Her symptoms worsened over time.

▪ Radiologic Findings

Sagittal gadolinium magnetic resonance imaging (MRI) of the thoracic spine demonstrates a T8–T10 enhancing intradural extramedullary lesion (**Fig. 64–1**).

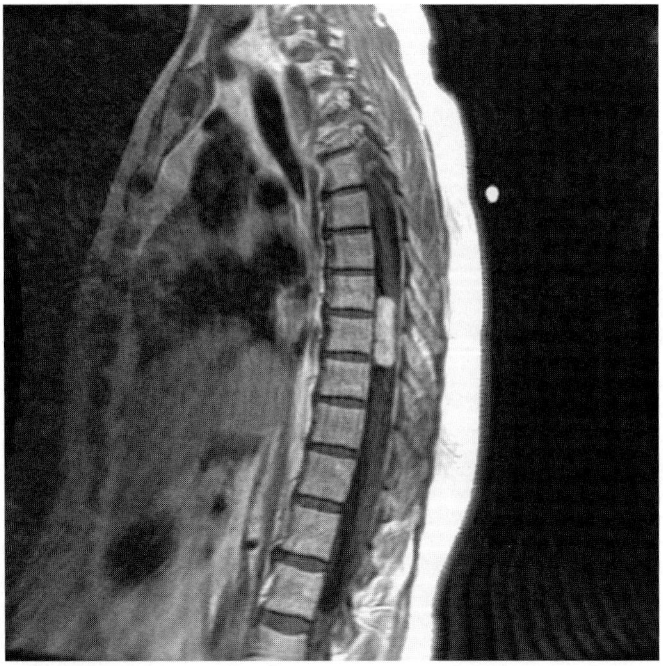

FIGURE 64–1 Gadolinium-enhancing thoracic intradural extramedullary lesion as seen on thoracic MRI.

▪ Diagnosis

Thoracic meningioma

▪ Treatment

A thoracic laminectomy with microresection was done.

▪ Discussion

Spinal meningiomas encompass 25 to 40% of extramedullary primary spinal tumors, and are more prominent in middle-aged women. The mean time before diagnosis is about a year, and the most common complaint is paraparesis followed by radicular pain. A thoracic location is the most frequent, then cervical. An anterior or anterolateral location is slightly more common than a posterior or posterolateral location. The meningothelial subtype is the most popular.

Surgical resection usually results in improvement. The calcified component of the meningioma and the ventral component (if present) are the riskiest aspects of resection. In addition, extradural spinal meningiomas, although rare, are higher risk tumors. They are believed to arise from the segment of the nerve root where the arachnoid is in contact with the dura. These occur in younger male patients, and can be more aggressive.

A key element to a successful surgery is the use of microsurgical technique along with intraoperative neurophysiologic monitoring. Tumor resection should attempt devascularization along its dural attachment. Piecemeal resection is undertaken to avoid cord manipulation. The use of intraoperative ultrasound can optimize tumor localization.

SUGGESTED READING

Klekamp J, Samii M. Surgical results for spinal meningiomas. Surg Neurol 1999;52:552–562

65

Spinal Tumor

ASIM MAHMOOD

■ Presentation

A 60-year-old woman had gait difficulty and back pain. On examination, her reflexes were brisk and she had lost proprioception. Her symptoms were worse at night.

■ Radiologic Findings

An intramedullary lesion with an associated syrinx is noted on thoracic magnetic resonance imaging (MRI) (**Figs. 65–1** and **65–2**).

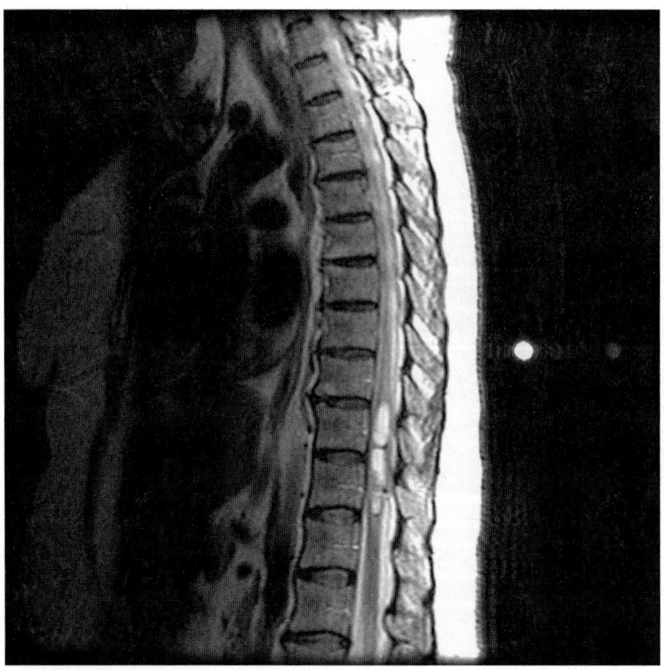

FIGURE 65–1 Sagittal MRI is notable for a thoracic intramedullary lesion with an associated syrinx.

■ Diagnosis

Pathology was diagnostic for a thoracic ependymoma

■ Treatment

A thoracic laminectomy for lesion excision with somatosensory evoked potential (SSEP) monitoring was done. Intraoperative photos display the tumor and the resection bed (**Figs. 65–3** and **65–4**).

■ Discussion

Ependymomas are glial tumors that arise from ependymal cells. In the spine, they usually affect adults. The most common spinal variant is the myxopapillary ependymoma of the conus and cauda equina. An important intraoperative difference between the other more commonly seen

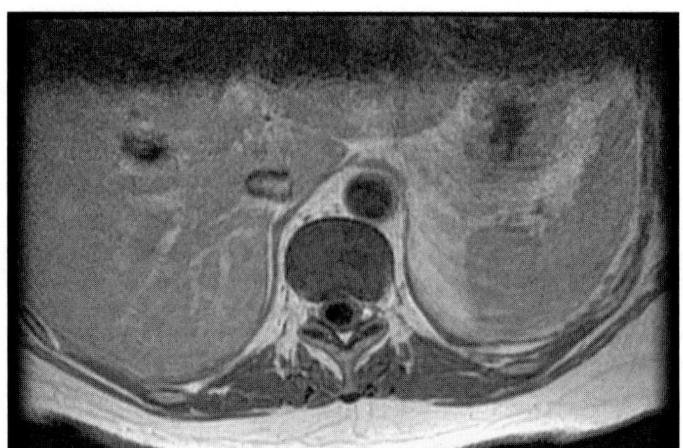

FIGURE 65–2 Axial MRI through the lesion.

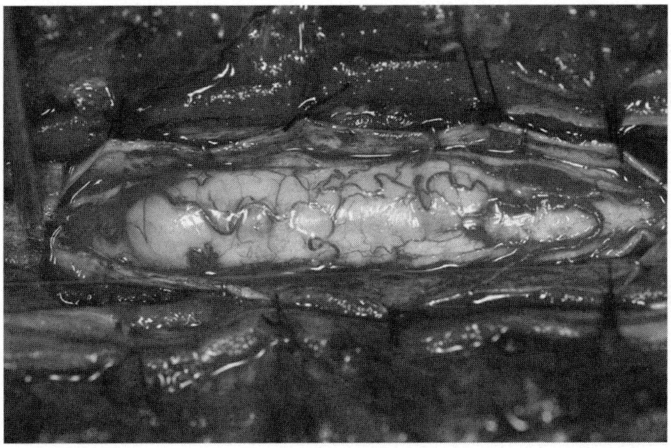

FIGURE 65–3 Intraoperative photo showing the dura opened and the spinal cord displacement by the tumor.

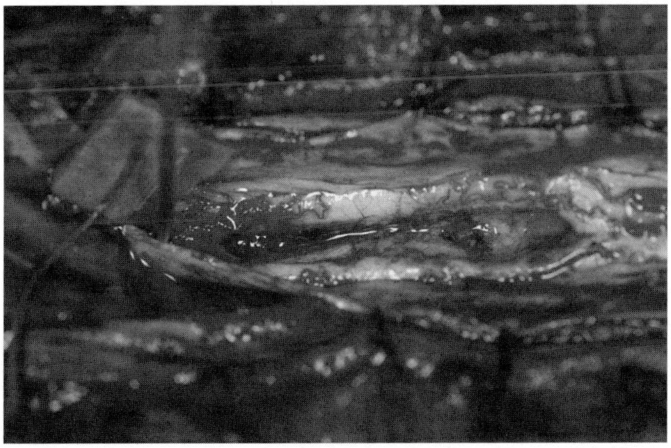

FIGURE 65–4 This intraoperative photo was taken at the resection.

intramedullary spinal tumor—the astrocytoma—is that the plane between the ependymoma and normal cord is well developed. Recurrence in the spine after a gross total resection is rare. The need for adjuvant treatment depends on tumor type and the totality of resection.

Intramedullary cystic dilatations are usually central in location and either lined with ependyma (hydromyelia) or not lined with ependyma (syringomyelia). These are also known as a syrinx, and can be either communicating or noncommunicating. A communicating syrinx is open to the obex or fourth ventricle and tends to be associated with Chiari I or II malformations. Noncommunicating dilatations may contain an amber or proteinaceous fluid and are associated with intramedullary tumors or are posttraumatic.

Ependymomas and hemangioblastomas are intramedullary tumors that present with cystic dilatations (**Figs. 65–5** and **65–6**). Tumor resection can also result in syrinx improvement; complete resection usually negates the need for additional syrinx-related procedures. Surgical

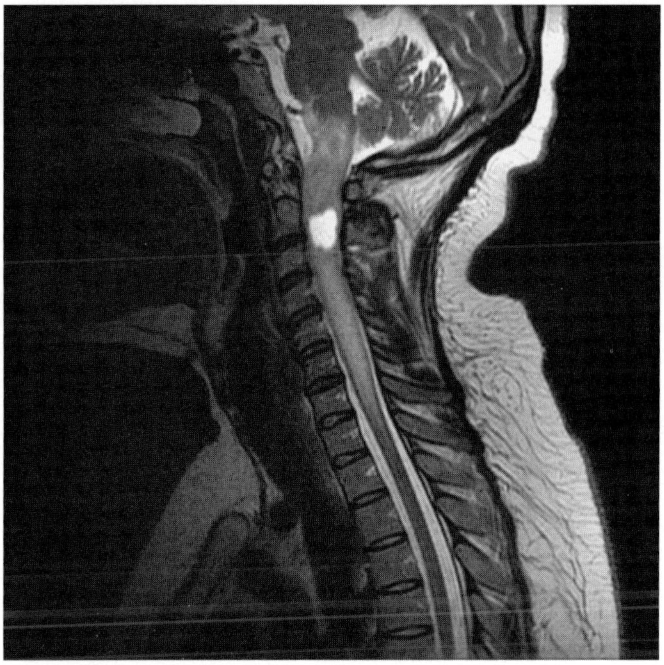

FIGURE 65–5 T2-weighted sagittal MRI of the cervical spine exhibiting an intramedullary ependymoma with a cystic component.

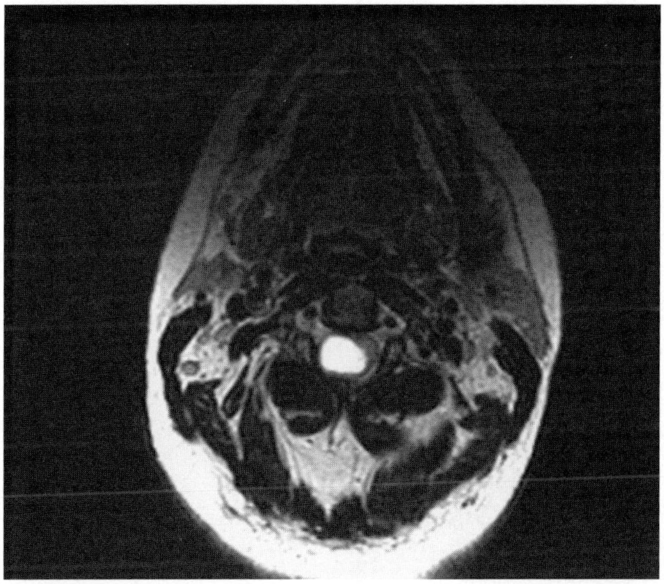

FIGURE 65–6 Axial MRI through the cystic area featured in **Fig. 65–5.**

resection requires precise microsurgical technique under neurophysiologic monitoring. Intraoperative ultrasound helps with tumor localization.

SUGGESTED READING

Hanbali F, Fourney DR, Marmor E, et al. Spinal cord ependymoma: a radical surgical resection and outcome. Neurosurgery 2002; 51:1162–1172

66

Lumbar Schwannoma

■ Presentation

A 48-year-old man complained of low back pain with radicular symptoms. He has no neurologic deficits. Computed tomography (CT) myelogram showed a complete block at the L4 level from a mass extending into the foramen.

■ Radiologic Findings

Magnetic resonance imaging (MRI) showed an intradural extramedullary lesion involving the lumbar roots at the L4 level (**Fig. 66–1**).

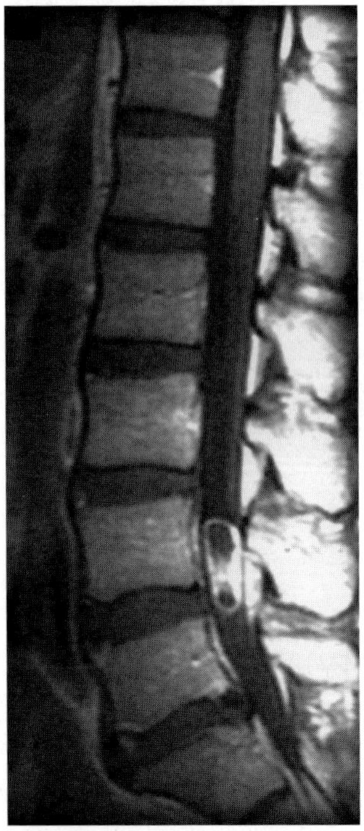

FIGURE 66–1 Gadolinium sagittal lumbar MRI with an intradural extramedullary mass extending into the foramen.

■ Pathology Findings and Diagnosis

Schwannoma without atypical features. Notice the Antoni A pattern, which is more compactly arranged than the looser Antoni B pattern (**Fig. 66–2**).

■ Treatment

The patient underwent L4 and L5 bilateral laminectomies for microsurgical resection of an intradural tumor. Given his gross total resection, recurrence is unlikely, but he will be followed with periodic MRI for the next couple of years.

■ Discussion

Tumors of the spine are classified into one of three compartments. Extradural tumors are usually metastatic.

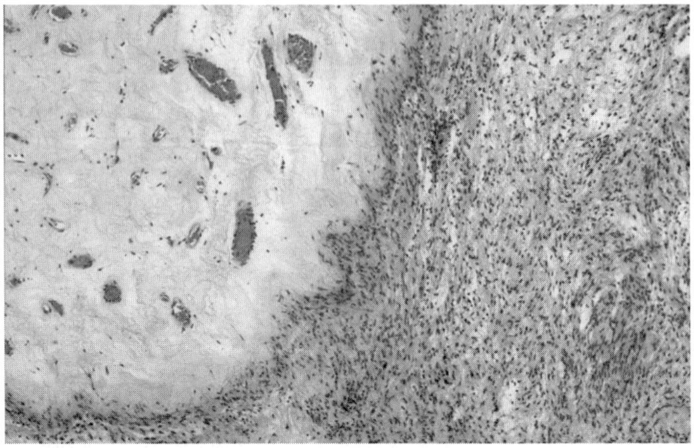

FIGURE 66–2 Pathology slide of schwannoma. Note the difference between the compact Antoni A pattern and the looser Antoni B pattern.

Another extradural tumor seen in practice is the multiple myeloma, or less commonly, primary bone tumors. Intradural extramedullary lesions include the nerve sheath tumors, meningiomas, or lipomas. Intramedullary tumors are the rarest, and include astrocytoma, ependymoma, and hemangioblastoma. In younger patients, one must also consider the possibility of drop metastases from a posterior fossa lesion.

Schwannomas originate from sensory nerve roots and are more easily delineated from their nerve roots than neurofibromas. This allows the possibility of removal without sacrificing the parent nerve root. Occasionally the lateral extension of this benign tumor necessitates a facetectomy for complete exposure, which in turn necessitates an additional fusion procedure. In this case, the tumor was easily accessed through laminectomies and no fusion was required.

Another consideration when operating on the intradural compartment of the lumbar spine is to ensure watertight closure of the dura. This can be done primarily and may also incorporate dural extenders and any of the biologic "glues" available. Careful dural closure is especially important when one takes into account the standing load of the lumbar spine.

If a schwannoma is totally resected, no adjuvant therapy is needed. Close radiographic monitoring is advisable for the first 2 years, or as dictated by the patient's clinical course. Notably, the addition of hardware can degrade postoperative imaging, and compromise serial scanning as a follow-up plan.

SUGGESTED READING

Celli P. Treatment of relevant nerve roots involved in nerve sheath tumors: removal or preservation? Neurosurgery 2002;51:684–692

67

Metastatic Spinal Cord Lesion

▪ Presentation

A 66-year-old man with non–small-cell lung cancer developed lower extremity weakness and incontinence over a period of days. He was paraparetic on examination, but did not have spine tenderness to percussion. A complete spine magnetic resonance imaging (MRI) did not show any cord compression.

▪ Radiologic Findings

Cervical MRI (**Fig. 67–1**) shows enlargement of the spinal cord by an intramedullary lesion.

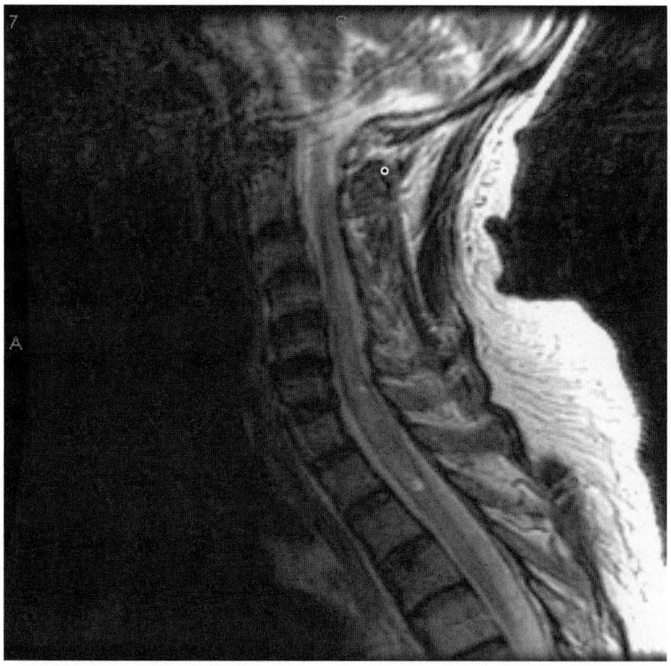

FIGURE 67–1 An intramedullary lesion is seen enlarging the cervical spinal cord on MRI.

▪ Diagnosis

Intramedullary metastatic spine lesion

▪ Treatment

Spinal radiation was given.

▪ Discussion

Although the most common intramedullary spinal cord lesions are astrocytoma, ependymoma, and hemangioblastoma, intramedullary metastases are on the rare end of the spectrum. Less than 1% of all spinal cord tumors can be categorized as such. Lung and breast are the most common primaries, but renal and gastrointestinal carcinomas have also contributed to the case report literature on cord metastases. One may also see drop metastases from primary brain lesions. Hemicord symptoms are not uncommonly described. Both surgery and radiation have been described with varied results.

SUGGESTED READING

Schiff D, O'Neill BP. Intramedullary spinal cord metastases: clinical features and treatment outcome. Neurology 1996;47:906–912

68

Sacral Lesion

■ Presentation

A 38-year-old man was troubled by lower extremity radiculopathies. Although he did not have incontinence, urinary frequency with decreased sensation in a right L5 to S3 distribution developed. An urgent workup was completed.

■ Radiologic Findings

A large, soft tissue density presacral lesion was seen on magnetic resonance imaging (MRI), displacing his pelvic structures (**Figs. 68–1** and **68–2**).

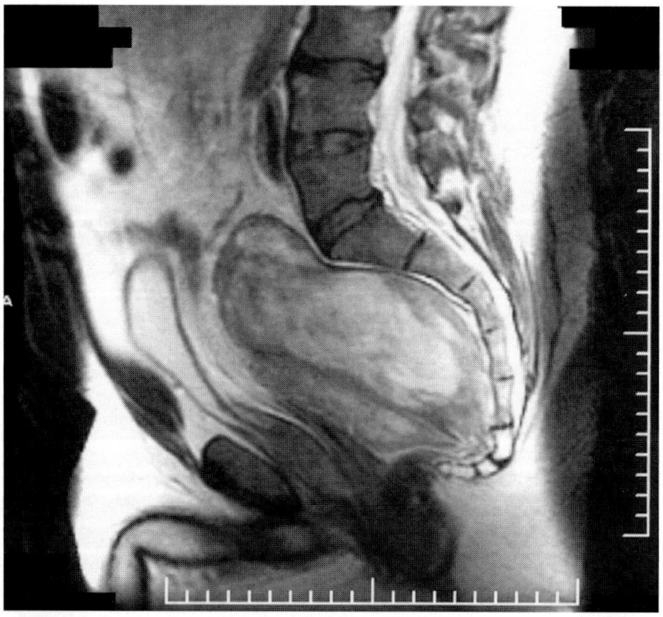

FIGURE 68–1 Sagittal MRI of the lumbosacral spine with a large presacral lesion.

■ Diagnosis

The results of pathology tests indicated a ganglioneuroma

■ Treatment

Through a combined transabdominal and transperianal approach, the tumor was resected. Electrophysiologic monitoring was utilized intraoperatively.

■ Discussion

Solid presacral tumors are usually malignant, and most frequently include primitive neuroectodermal tumors

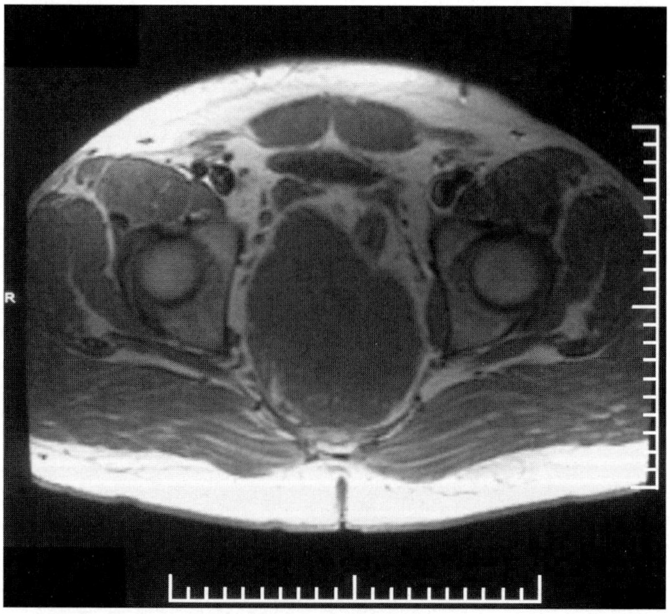

FIGURE 68–2 Axial MRI through the lesion.

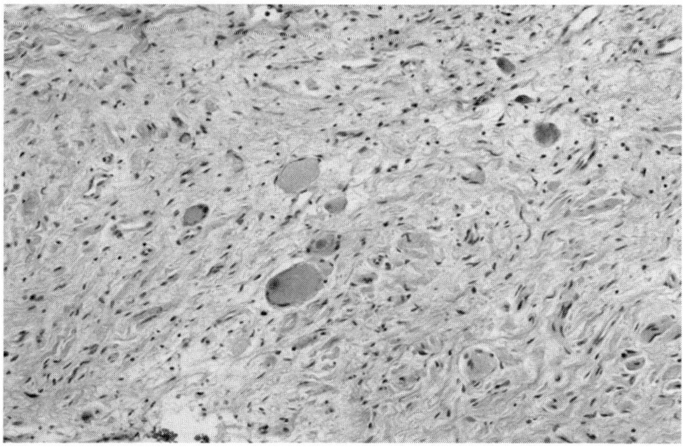

FIGURE 68–3 Ganglion cells.

(PNET) and sacrococcygeal teratomas. Enteric cysts and anterior sacral meningoceles are among cystic presacral lesions. Congenital lesions usually involve a bony defect and urologic abnormalities.

This patient had an even more rare presacral mass. Ganglioneuromas are benign and usually seen in the posterior mediastinum or retroperitoneum. One will see a proliferation of Schwann cells and ganglion cells under the microscope (**Fig. 68–3**). Surgical extirpation is a cure.

Different surgical approaches, both open and laparoscopic, are used for these tumors. In this case, the tumor size was formidable, and a transabdominal transperianal approach was the most advantageous. Familiarity with the approach and preoperative discussion with the approaching surgeon will result in a successful team resection.

SUGGESTED READING

Kohler C, Kuhne-Heid R, Klemm P, Tozzi R, Schneider A. Resection of a presacral ganglioneurofibroma by laparoscopy. Surg Endosc 2003;17:1499

69

Recurrent Sacral Tumor

■ Presentation

A 44-year-old man complained of recurrent sacral pain, sexual dysfunction, and radicular symptoms. He had previous resection of a sacral mass, followed by radiation and chemotherapy. He was neurologically intact.

■ Radiologic Findings

A large heterogeneous sacral mass with a high T2 signal intensity is noted on a lumbosacral magnetic resonance imaging (MRI) (**Figs. 69–1** and **69–2**).

■ Diagnosis

Sacral liposarcoma

■ Treatment

A combined transabdominal, transperineal, and posterior approach was done for resection with neurophysiologic monitoring.

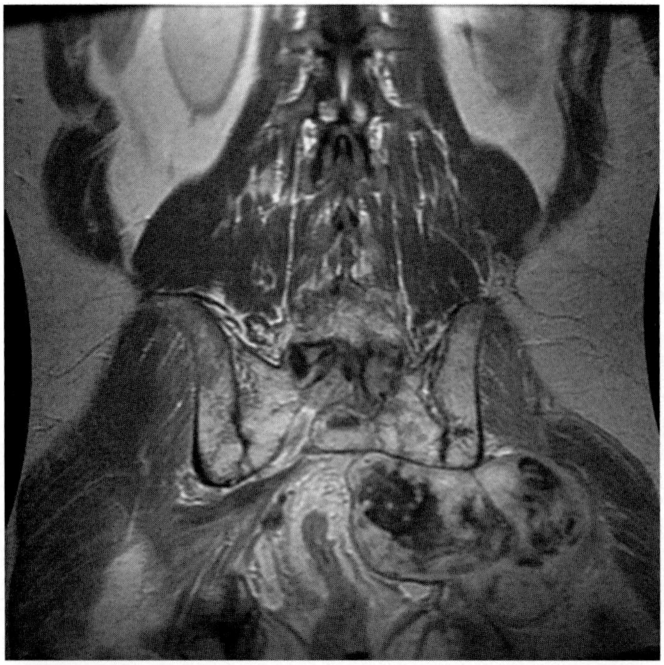

FIGURE 69–1 A large heterogenous sacral mass with a high T2 signal intensity is noted on a coronal lumbosacral MRI.

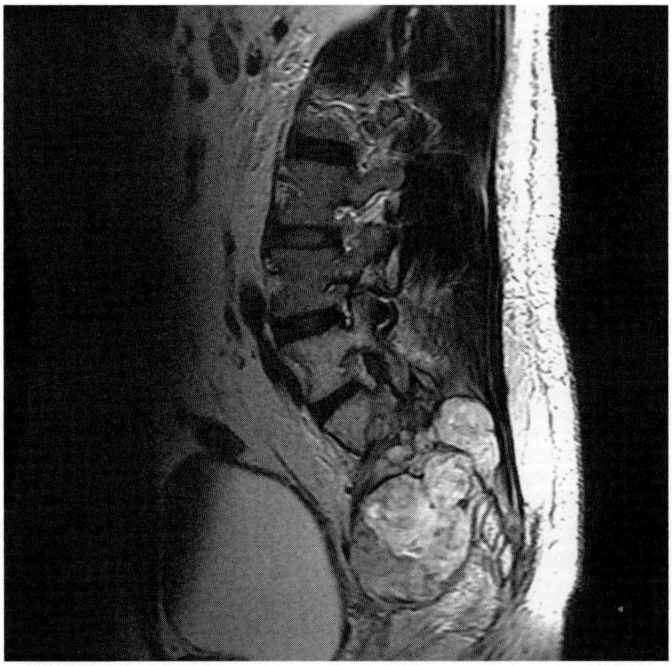

FIGURE 69–2 The same lesion is noted on a sagittal MRI through the region.

■ Discussion

Although chordomas are a common tumor in this location, the differential includes liposarcoma, teratoma, malignant fibrous histiocytoma, desmoid, leiomyosarcoma, and lymphoma. The fatty, noncalcific components of this patient's liposarcoma helped in differentiating this tumor radiologically. Myxoid, well-differentiated, and pleomorphic liposarcoma subtypes exist. It usually is diagnosed in men in their 50s to 70s, and has an overall 5-year survival rate of 30%.

Chordomas are a rare malignant midline tumor, most commonly seen at the cranial and caudal ends of the notochord remnants. Chordomas are derived from notochord cell rests, and usually occur in men ages 55 to 65. Chordomas are destructive bone masses with soft tissue invasion. Microscopically, physaliphorous cells (large, vacuolated cytoplasmic cells) are present. The treatment is usually a combination of surgery and radiation, and prognosis is more favorable if the resection is complete. Contamination of the surgical area with tumor increases the local recurrence rate. The 5-year survival rate is 50%, and all chordomas will metastasize later in their course.

Surgery in the retroperitoneal and sacral area has many potential complications. Vascular, visceral, nerve root, and plexal injury are a risk. The tumor and its bony and soft tissue invasion can lead to a high blood loss during resection. Wound healing in this area and the proximity of the wound to the perineum and anus can increase the infection rate. In addition, with an aggressive resection, lumbosacral and sacroiliac stability may be in question. The use of prostheses and the variety of systems available for lumbopelvic and sacroiliac fixation are helpful in restoring stability and sagittal balance.

SUGGESTED READING

Boriani S, Weinstein JN, Biagini R. Primary bone tumors of the spine. Terminology and surgical staging. Spine 1997;22:1036–1044

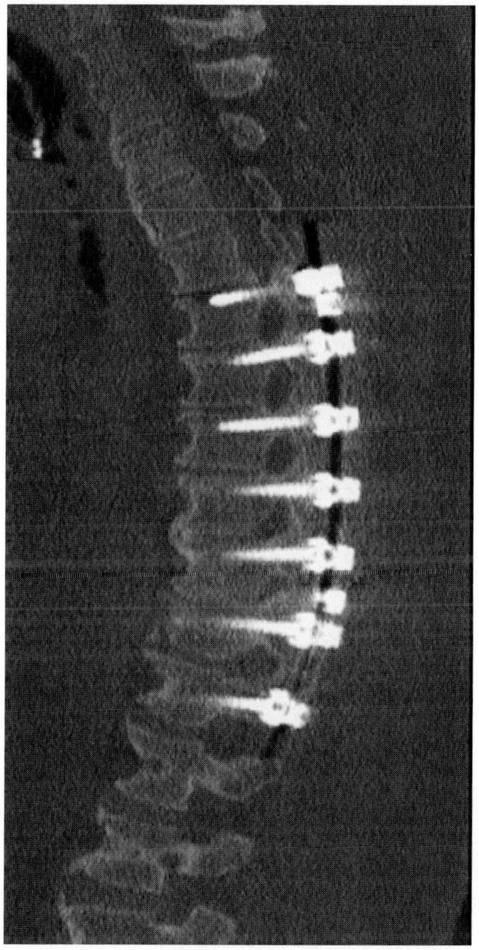

FIGURE 71–2 Sagittal reconstructed CT of the postoperative construct.

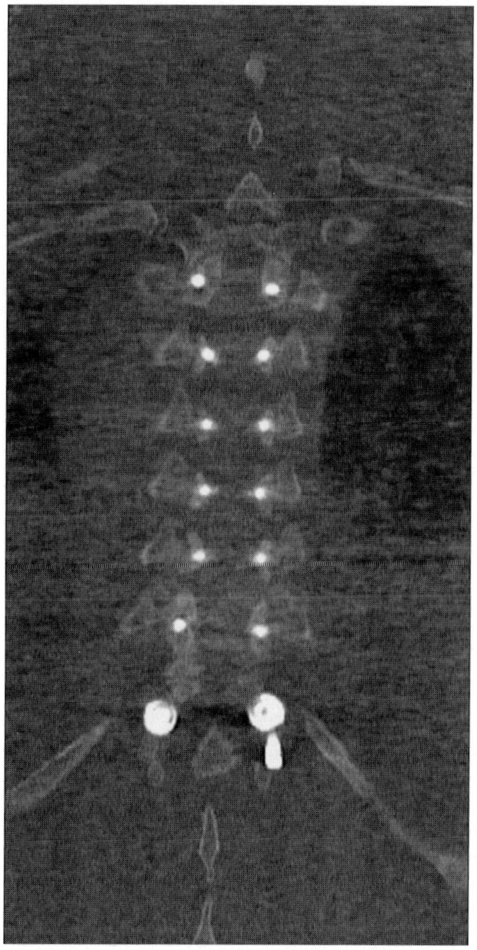

FIGURE 71–3 Coronal reconstructed CT of the thoracic pedicle screws.

Persistent, severe axial pain necessitated operative intervention for this patient. Multiple bone biopsies and laboratory data proved the infection was resolved preoperatively. As he developed a solid fusion, his pain subsided.

SUGGESTED READING

Hadjipavlou AG, Mader JT, Necessary JT, Muffoletto AJ. Hematogenous pyogenic spinal infections and their surgical management. Spine 2000;25:1668–1679

72

Pott's Disease

■ Presentation

A 68-year-old woman had Pott's disease as a child, and underwent several corrective lumbar procedures. She presented with progressive pain and gait and bowel/bladder dysfunction.

■ Radiologic Findings

Preoperatively, spinal magnetic resonance imaging (MRI) showed severe compression of the dural sac with an abnormal kyphoscoliosis at L2–L3 by a mass likely derived from her previous granulomatous inflammation (**Figs. 72–1** and **72–2**). In addition, her lumbosacral spine is significantly spondylotic with a previous fusion at L4–L5 noted.

■ Diagnosis

Postinfectious deformity

■ Treatment

Using a bilateral transpedicular approach and redo laminectomy, a ventral extradural mass was encountered. This consisted of calcified, caseating material (**Fig. 72–3**). This was removed piecemeal to restore the spinal canal. No fusion was needed, because she was autofused from her previous disease.

■ Discussion

The most common site of extrapulmonary involvement of tuberculosis (TB) is the thoracolumbar spine. TB of the spine is called Pott's disease, and the infection first affects the vertebral body and then spreads to the disc space. Specifically, the anterior aspect of the vertebral body adjacent to the subchondral plate is the initial spinal area affected. Although relatively uncommon

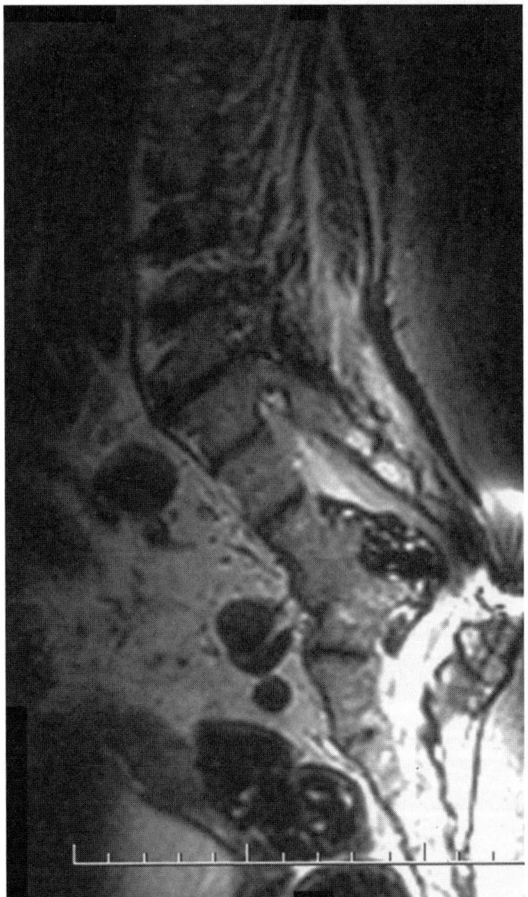

FIGURE 72–1 Sagittal MRI shows L2–L3 kyphoscoliosis.

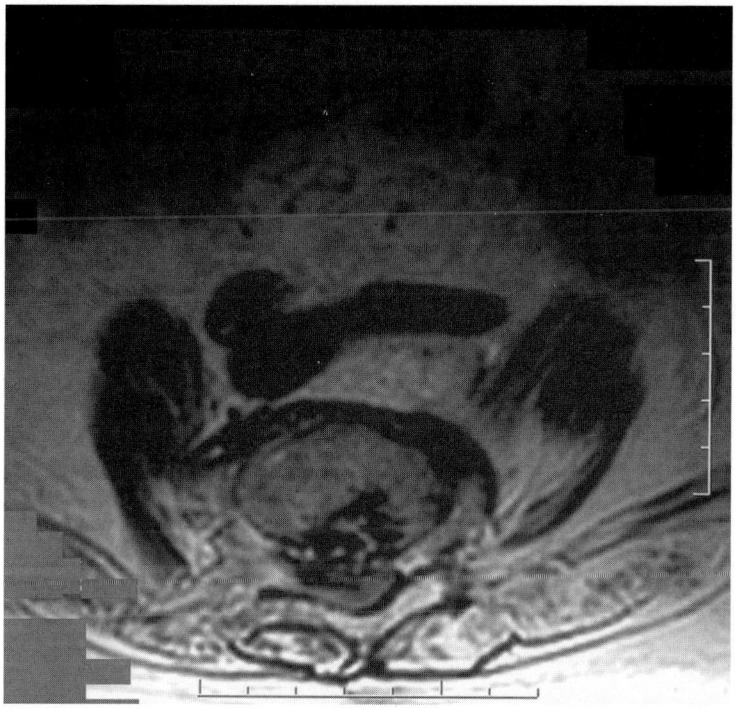

FIGURE 72–2 Axial MRI through the area of maximal deformity.

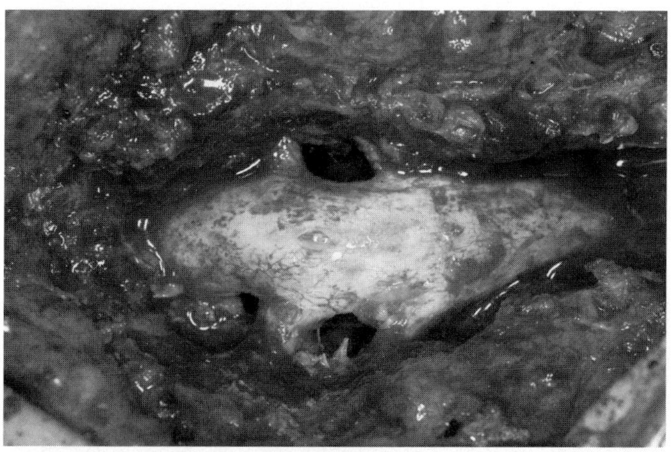

FIGURE 72–3 Intraoperative photo.

in the modern Western world, Pott's disease can cause a painful and progressive deformity. HIV-positive and immunocompromised patients are at higher risk. Most of these patients autofuse from the pathology and are left with neurologic deficit.

Diagnostic studies of choice are sedimentation rate, TB skin testing, needle biopsy if surgery is not planned (although there is a high rate of false negatives), and serial imaging with x-ray, computed tomography (CT), and the gold standard, MRI. An extraspinal source of infection should be sought out and treated. Once the diagnosis is established, the treatment is medical with surgical debridement and fusion if needed, and a brace to prevent progressive deformity. Progressive bone destruction leads to vertebral collapse and kyphosis, and the spinal canal can be further narrowed by abscesses, granulation tissues, or dural invasion. Spread can extend to the musculature and surrounding soft tissue.

Depending on the resistance, a three- or four-drug regimen should be used for a total of 12 months, with additional drugs during the first 2 months. Isoniazid, rifampin, and pyrazinamide are the core of the drug regimens. Indications for surgical intervention in addition to drug treatment are acute neurologic deficit or spinal deformity with instability. Other indications are no response to medical therapy or a nondiagnostic biopsy.

SUGGESTED READING

Dharmalingam M. Tuberculosis of the spine—the Sabah experience. Epidemiology, treatment and results. Tuberculosis (Edinb) 2004;84:24–28

73

Intramedullary Cervical Lesion

■ Presentation

A 61-year-old man developed increasing quadriparesis and spasticity. He had a remote history of foreign travel.

■ Radiologic Findings

A T2-weighted cervical magnetic resonance imaging (MRI) is remarkable for a loculated, intramedullary hyperintense lesion that is widening the cord at C2 (**Figs. 73–1** and **73–2**).

■ Diagnosis

Intramedullary cysticercosis

■ Treatment

Surgical drainage and excision with microsurgical technique and neurophysiologic monitoring were done.

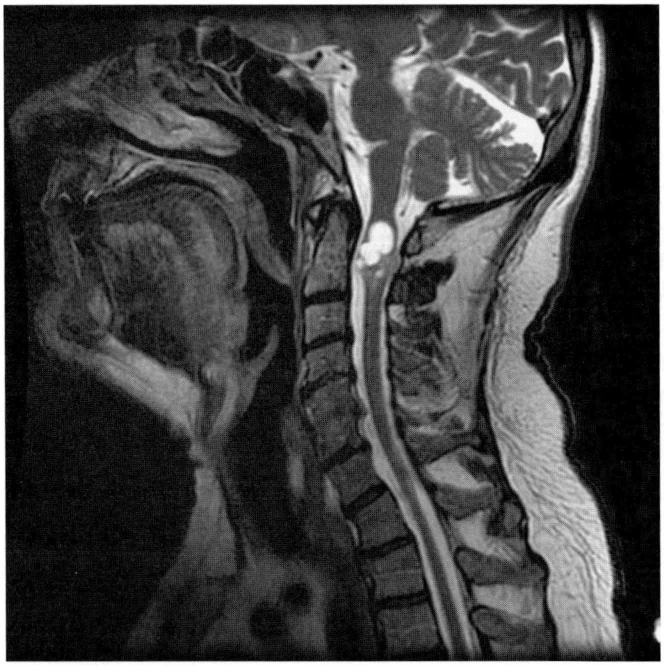

FIGURE 73–1 A loculated C2 lesion expands the cord prominently on a cervical MRI.

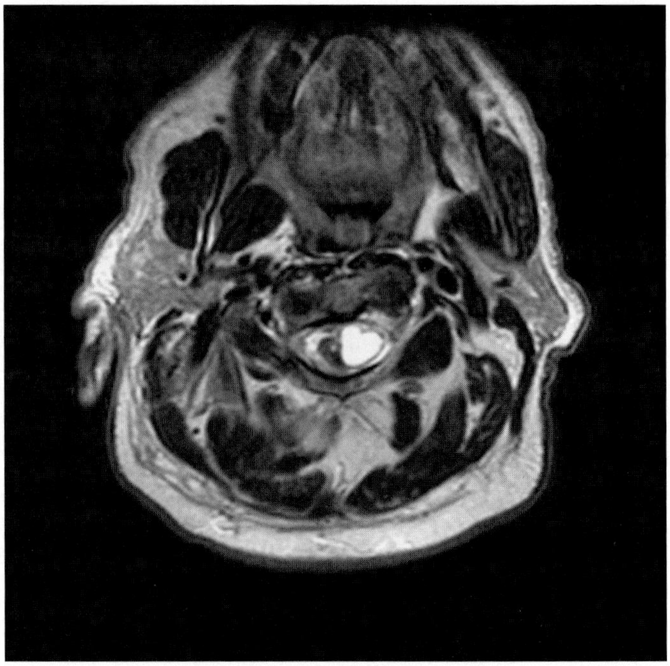

FIGURE 73–2 This hyperintense intramedullary lesion is again visualized on an axial slice through the area of interest.

■ Discussion

Intramedullary cystic lesions are rare occurrences. They can be related to various pathologies, including neoplastic, infectious, inflammatory, demyelinating, degenerative, vascular, or even radiation-induced causes. Parasites are lesser known causes of intramedullary cystic lesions. Yet, these infections of the central nervous system (cysticercosis and hydatid cysts) are endemic in certain areas of the world.

Neurocysticercosis occurs with some frequency in Mexico, Central and South America, Africa, the Far East (India and China), and in California as well. Spinal neurocysticercosis is a rare but debilitating form of the disease. It accounts for less than 1% of reported cases of the disease. Subarachnoid cervical spine neurocysticercosis is the most common site by far and is a likely result of the ventricular to subarachnoid migration of the pathogen. Intramedullary spinal neurocysticercosis is even rarer, and is mostly reported in the thoracic cord. It is postulated to occur there because of the nature of the spinal cord vascular supply.

The presentation of the spinal cord disease depends on its location and progression, with paraplegia and quadriplegia being the most common signs. Early on, progressive myelopathy with bowel/bladder dysfunction is common. Brown-Séquard syndrome (hemicord syndrome) has also been reported. Diagnosis is based on clinical, radiographic, and serologic studies, but the disease should be considered in patients with severe progressive neurologic deficit and a history of exposure to endemic areas. Imaging of the entire neuraxis is needed. Treatment of spinal cord cysticercosis often requires surgical intervention to extirpate the lesion or lesions and decompress the cord. The patients then have to take anticysticercosis drug therapy, such as flubendazole, albendazole, and praziquantel. The use of dexamethasone has been advocated in the acute phase to halt the progress of neurologic deficit.

SUGGESTED READING

Wei GZ, Li CJ, Meng JM, Ding MC. Cysticercosis of the central nervous system: a clinical study of 1400 cases. Chin Med J (Engl) 1988; 101:493–500

■ PART VI ■

Congenital

74

Klippel-Feil Spine

■ Presentation

A 41-year-old woman with Klippel-Feil syndrome complained of chronic neck and upper extremity pain, radiating into both hands. This improved with shaking her hands out, and was worsened by repetitive movements. On physical examination, she had the typical aborted neck of these patients, and her examination uncovered a positive Phalen's sign bilaterally.

■ Radiologic Findings

X-ray and magnetic resonance imaging (MRI) of the cervical spine show the classical fusion of cervical vertebral bodies and basilar invagination, without cord compression (**Figs. 74–1** and **74–2**).

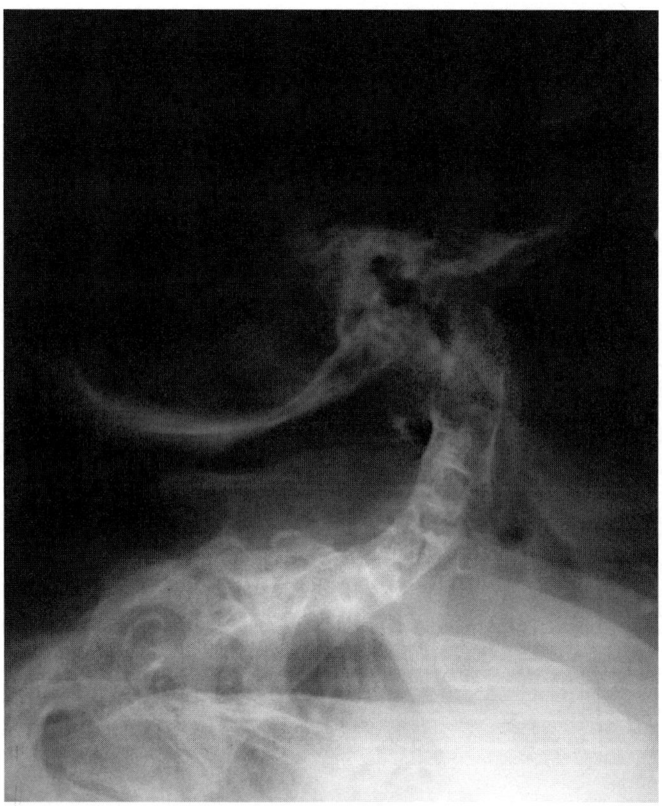

FIGURE 74–1 X-ray of the cervical spine shows autofusion over multiple segments.

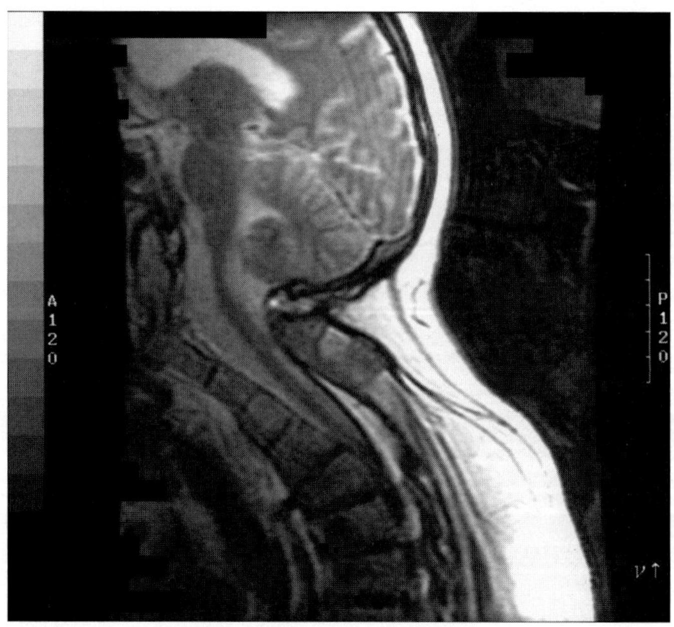

FIGURE 74–2 MRI of the cervical spine again showing multisegmental fusion and an open cervical canal.

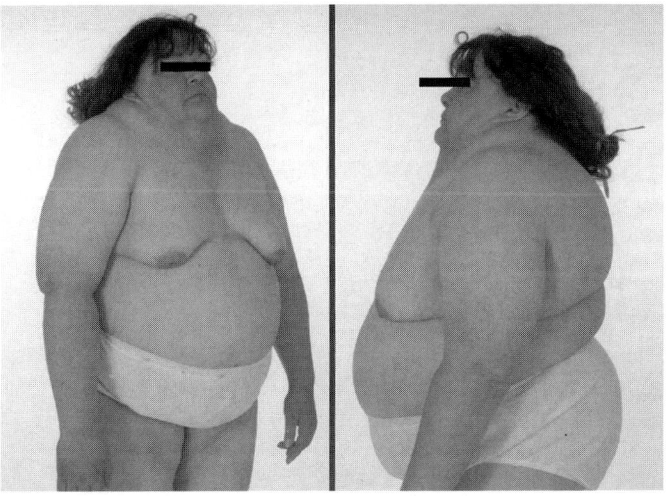

FIGURE 74–3 This patient has the typical morphology of Klippel-Feil Syndrome.

■ Diagnosis

Carpal tunnel syndrome

■ Treatment

The patient was sent for electromyogram (EMG), which indicated carpal tunnel syndrome bilaterally. She responded well to a 6-week trial of wrist support and anti-inflammatory medication.

■ Discussion

Klippel-Feil syndrome patients usually have a low dorsal hairline, congenital fusion of cervical vertebrae with subsequent decreased range of motion, and scoliosis. They typically present with a triad of neck pain, limited cervical range of motion, and deformity. Torticollis, webbed neck, and facial asymmetry are frequent findings (**Fig. 74–3**). Even in patients with the complex cervical pathology of Klippel-Feil syndrome, the peripheral nerve examination may uncover the root of their presenting problem. Classical carpal tunnel history and examination findings, such as a positive Phalen's sign, worsening with repetitive movements, and improvement with shaking out the hand, can be verified with EMG. EMG is positive in 70% of carpal tunnel cases. The patient was treated conservatively and improved without surgery.

SUGGESTED READING

Tracy MR, Dormans JP, Kusumi K. Klippel-Feil syndrome: clinical features and current understanding of etiology. Clin Orthop 2004;424:183–190

75

Klippel-Feil Syndrome

■ Presentation

A 46-year-old woman with Klippel-Feil syndrome presented with gait instability and dysesthetic arm pain. She had some hand weakness. Magnetic resonance imaging (MRI) of the C-spine was notable for stenosis, mostly at the foramen magnum, and autofusion of the first five cervical vertebral bodies.

■ Radiologic Findings

Cervical x-ray taken postoperatively shows occipitocervical fusion instrumentation and vertebral body findings typical of Klippel-Feil syndrome (**Fig. 75–1**).

■ Diagnosis

Upper cervical stenosis in a patient with Klippel-Feil syndrome

■ Treatment

The patient had a suboccipital craniectomy and C1 laminectomy with occipitocervical fusion.

■ Discussion

Klippel-Feil remains a fascinating and multifaceted syndrome. The classic triad is a low posterior hairline, short neck, and limitation of neck motion due to fused cervical vertebrae. Additional findings include possible basilar impression, atlanto-occipital fusion, facial palsy, scoliosis, a raised scapula (Sprengel's deformity), synkinesis, absence of a kidney, and deafness.

The most commonly observed pathology is in the cervical spine. The involved vertebrae are typically wide and flat, with an absent or hypoplastic, immobile disc space. Often, three to five vertebrae are fused together, putting additional stress on the adjacent segments, causing accelerated degeneration. This can cause spinal canal compromise. Patients usually present with neck

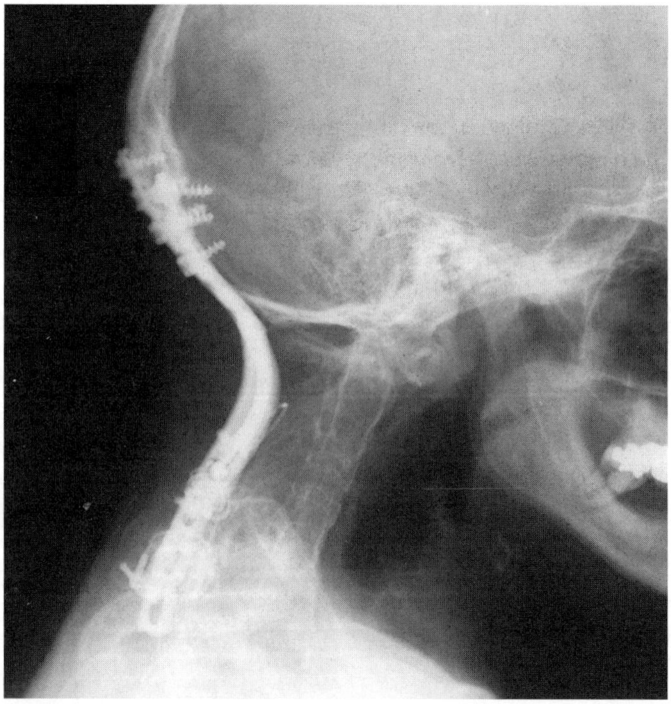

FIGURE 75–1 Cervical x-ray shows the patient's subaxial autofusion augmented by an occipitocervical fusion with rods and sublaminar wiring.

pain and neurologic compromise. One should also examine the lower cranial nerves and assess for other symptoms of cervicomedullary junction compromise.

This patient's presentation was typical. She benefited from decompression of her stenosis with fusion. Of note, it is important to keep in mind that the previous autofusion of her vertebral bodies plus the iatrogenically imposed occipitocervical fusion will put great stress on the hardware, as her neck motion is limited. For this reason, these patients are at greater risk for hardware failure.

The use of a naturally curved structural autograft, such as a rib graft, can be the optimal graft substitute to accommodate the challenging contour of the craniocervical junction. The choice of grafting material is key to ensure a solid arthrodesis in these high-risk patients.

SUGGESTED READING

Theiss SM, Smith MD, Winter RB. The long term follow up of patients with Klippel-Feil syndromes and congenital scoliosis. Spine 1997;22:1219–1222

76

Cervical Rib

■ Presentation

A 50-year-old man was troubled by a recent onset of arm pain and numbness. He had no neurologic deficit. Mild cervical spondylosis was seen on magnetic resonance imaging (MRI).

■ Radiologic Findings

An anteroposterior (AP) C-spine x-ray is remarkable for the presence of a cervical rib (**Fig. 76–1**).

■ Diagnosis

Thoracic outlet syndrome

■ Treatment

A course of conservative therapy with pain control and physical therapy was initiated, and the patient will make follow-up visits to the clinic.

■ Discussion

Thoracic outlet syndrome is a controversial diagnosis that refers to the myriad of symptoms caused by compression of the brachial plexus, subclavian vein, or subclavian artery. Brachial plexus compression (C8 and T1) occurs most frequently and predominantly in females. In addition to medial arm and fourth and fifth digit pain, cold intolerance, headache, and fine motor weakness can occur with neurologic compression. Venous compression manifests as a painful, edematous arm, and arterial compression causes claudication, arm pallor, and pain. In addition, the latter patient will have lower blood pressure in the affected arm.

Often the physical examination is normal. Most provocative tests, like Adson's maneuver, are not very reliable, although asking the patient to abduct his arms 90 degrees from the thorax, flex his elbows, and rapidly open and close his hands for 3 minutes can reproduce thoracic outlet symptoms. On radiologic imaging, a

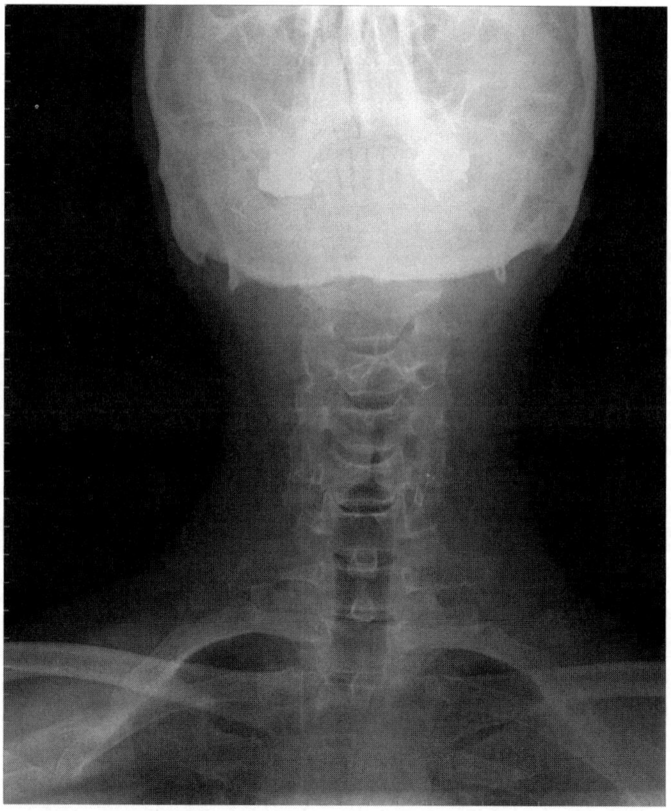

FIGURE 76–1 AP cervical x-ray with cervical rib.

cervical rib, elongation of the C7 transverse process, or a congenital fibromuscular band may be noted. The anterior and middle scalene muscles may also be the source of compression. There is some evidence that repetitive activity may play a part in this syndrome.

X-ray, arteriogram and venogram, or color flow duplex scanning may be employed for diagnosis. The cervical spine should be worked up with an MRI or myelogram. Electromyography and nerve conduction studies can be helpful.

A vascular etiology of thoracic outlet syndrome requires more urgent intervention, especially if there is evidence of ischemia or emboli. Anticoagulation, thrombectomy, or surgical decompression of the offending structure may be used depending on the cause. For neurologic presentations of thoracic outlet syndrome, an initial conservative approach with pain control, therapy, and behavior modification is utilized. Although surgical decompression may be used in patients who fail months of conservative therapy, the success rate is fairly disappointing, with an up to 60% failure to relieve symptoms in some series.

SUGGESTED READING

McGillicuddy JE. Cervical radiculopathy, entrapment neuropathy, and thoracic outlet syndrome: how to differentiate? J Neurosurg Spine 2004;1:179–187

77

Ankylosing Hyperostosis of Forestier and Rotes-Querol

■ Presentation

This 69-year-old man fell forward 6 months ago and began complaining of neck pain. He remains neurologically intact and without pain.

■ Radiologic Findings

C-spine lateral x-ray demonstrates diffuse ankylosing hyperostosis with ossifications involving the anterior aspect of the spine. The osteophytic bridge is disrupted at C2–C3 and C4–C5 (**Fig. 77–1**). The patient does not move on flexion extension films, and his alignment is intact.

■ Diagnosis

Diffuse idiopathic skeletal hyperostosis (DISH)

■ Treatment

Because there is no translational instability, subluxation, cord signal changes on magnetic resonance imaging (MRI), or other evidence of misalignment, and the patient is pain free, his collar was discontinued. His spine is stable after a fall 6 months ago.

■ Discussion

DISH is an ossifying disease of unknown etiology that affects ~10% of patients in the sixth decade of life. It is characterized by "flowing" calcifications and "claw" spurring of the anterolateral aspects of the involved vertebrae. DISH tends to affect the lumbar spine, usually at the L4 level. End-plate osteophytes and disc collapse are seen, and patients report low back pain. The cervical spine is also affected and is often an incidental finding or thought to be the etiology of dysphagia, and less often, myelopathy.

Differentiating DISH of the lumbar spine from degenerative stenosis can be nuanced. Leroux et al (1992) have

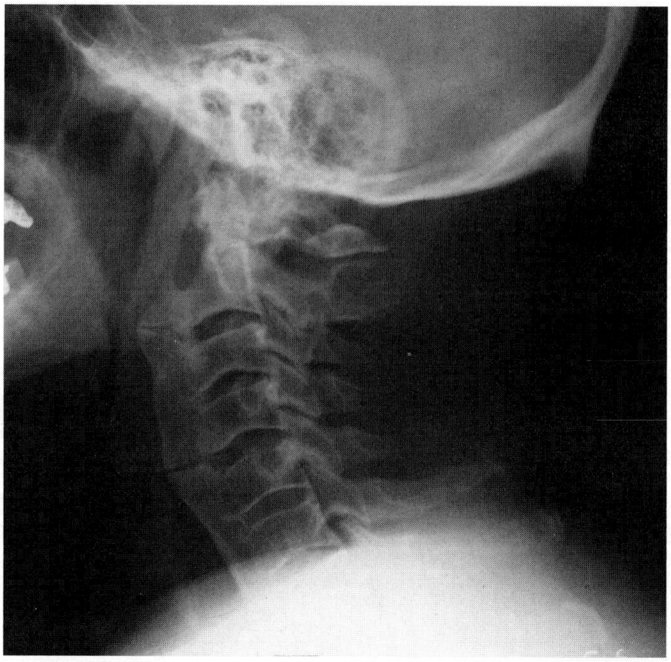

FIGURE 77–1 Lateral C-spine x-ray displays a classical picture of the osteophytic bridging seen in DISH.

established the following criteria as indicative for DISH: anterior or posterior lateral margin osseous proliferation, proliferation of the nonarticular aspects of the posterior apophysis, and ossification of the posterior articular capsule and posterior ligaments.

Our patient would have been a candidate for surgical resection if his osteophytes had symptomatic mass effect—either as a myelopathy or dysphagia. His disrupted osteophytic ridge is from previous injury, painless, and stable on dynamic studies. No further treatment is needed, but future radiologic follow-up would be prudent.

SUGGESTED READINGS

Leroux JL, Legeran P, Moniliner L, Laroche M. Stenosis of the lumbar spinal canal in vertebral ankylosing hyperostosis. Spine 1992;17:1213–1218

Mader R. Clinical manifestations of diffuse idiopathic skeletal hyperostosis of the cervical spine. Semin Arthritis Rheum 2002; 32:130–135

78

Fibrous Dysplasia

■ Presentation

A 67-year-old woman complained of upper neck pain worsened by neck extension, radiating into her left suboccipital region. Objectively, she has no focal neurologic deficit and a mild decrease in cervical range of motion.

■ Radiologic Findings

Computed tomography (CT) and magnetic resonance imaging (MRI) of the cervical spine demonstrated a destructive bony lesion involving the inferior part of C2, C1, and the clivus (**Figs. 78–1** and **78–2**).

■ Diagnosis

Skeletal dysplasia

■ Treatment

The patient was presented with four treatment options: (1) observation with medication, (2) biopsy, (3) posterior

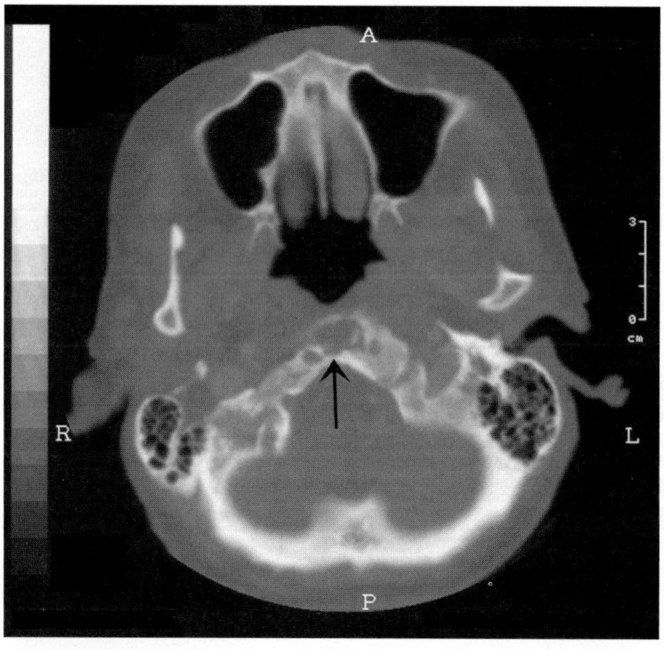

FIGURE 78–1 CT showing destructive bony lesion of C2.

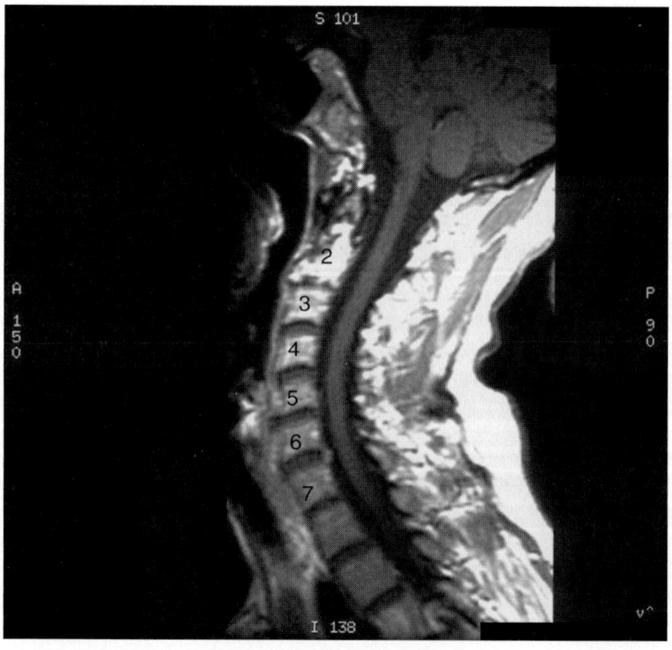

FIGURE 78–2 MRI showing lesion affecting C1, C2, and the clivus.

upper cervical fusion, and (4) vertebroplasty. She has similar lesions in her right arm and pelvis.

■ Discussion

The spine can be affected by numerous connective tissue syndromes that share a unifying theme. Thematically, they are metabolic diseases caused by a symptomatic defect in skeletal development. The matrix of the cartilage or the bone, or both, is affected. Deformity, instability, and stenosis of the spine can result. Examples of such skeletal dysplasias include achondroplasia, osteogenesis imperfecta, mucopolysaccharidoses, and diastrophic dysplasia.

Certain dysplasias share presentation specifics. Cervical kyphosis is commonly seen in Larsen's syndrome and diastrophic dysplasia. Thoracic and thoracolumbar kyphosis are mostly seen in achondroplasia, whereas scoliosis is seen in diastrophic and metatropic dysplasia. Foramen magnum stenosis is seen in almost all achondroplastic infants. This causes neurologic deficit, and, in severe cases, sleep apnea.

Although there are no treatment rules for this class of disorders, there are some common guidelines. If there is atlantoaxial instability of over 8 mm of translational movement on flexion-extension x-ray, a fusion should be seriously considered. Similarly, progressive thoracic kyphosis or kyphosis greater than 50 degrees should be assessed for stabilization. The presence of other comorbidities, the natural history of certain subtypes, and patient and family input into the treatment plan are important decision-making components.

SUGGESTED READING

Lachman RS. Neurologic abnormalities in the skeletal dysplasias: a clinical and radiological perspective. Am J Med Genet 1997; 69:33–43

79

Diastematomyelia

■ Presentation

A 59-year-old man presented with progressive kyphoscoliotic deformity of the thoracolumbar spine. He was neurologically intact. Further investigation found diastematomyelia.

■ Radiologic Findings

The patient's T2-weighted sagittal and axial thoracic magnetic resonance imaging (MRI) had a split cord malformation (**Figs. 79–1** and **79–2**).

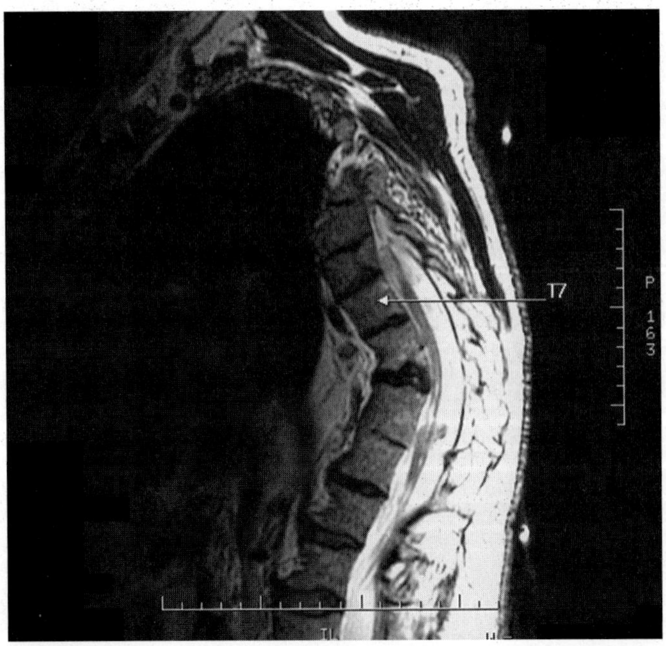

FIGURE 79–1 Sagittal thoracic MRI demonstrates diastematomyelia.

■ Diagnosis

Split cord malformation type II

■ Treatment

He had a thoracic laminectomy with removal of an intradural spur and cord untethering and segmental fusion, as demonstrated in pre– and post–spur removal intraoperative pictures (**Fig. 79–3**).

■ Discussion

Diastematomyelia is a spinal dysraphic state resulting in congenital splitting of a segment of the spinal canal.

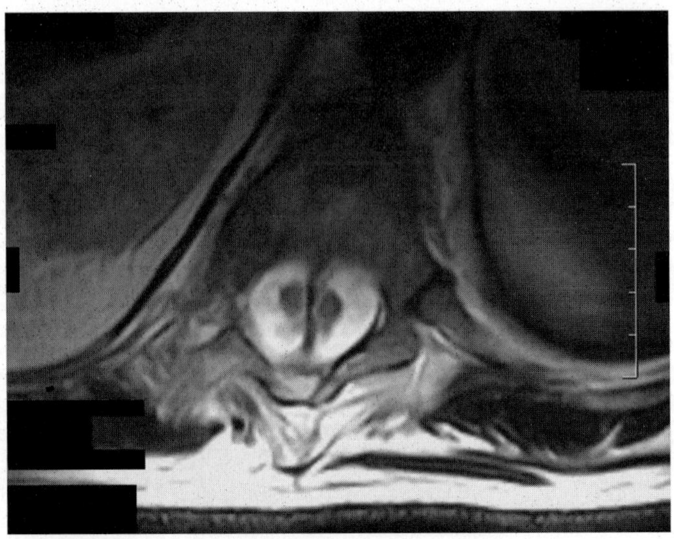

FIGURE 79–2 Axial MRI demonstrates diastematomyelia, with a bony ridge entering a single dural sac.

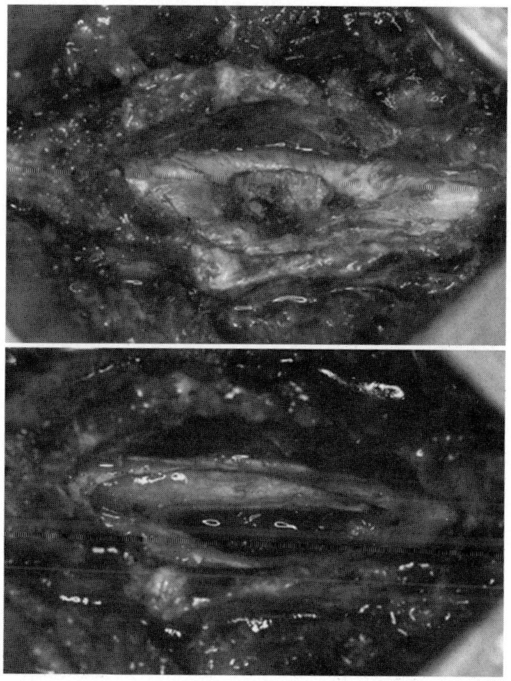

FIGURE 79–3 Intraoperative photo displaying the median septum prior to its removal (top) and then after its resection (bottom).

The split can be caused by a cartilaginous or fibrous barrier. In type I, the hemicords each have their own separate dural sac, and in type II both hemicords are housed in the same sac. The two hemicords reunite immediately caudad to the median barrier, creating a cord tethering. The cord is then at risk for traction injury after a spinal hyperflexion maneuver. Patients usually present with symptoms after being in a hyperflexion position (childbirth, motor vehicle crash, gymnastics) or during a growth spurt.

This disorder is more prevalent in females and often affects the thoracolumbar spine. Asymmetry of a limb (**Fig. 79–4**), orthopedic foot deformities, or pes cavus are earlier forms of presentation. Neurologic presentations are more prevalent in adolescence or adulthood and are characterized by back pain, dysesthesia, perineal pain, spastic paraparesis, neuropathic bladder, or an atonic

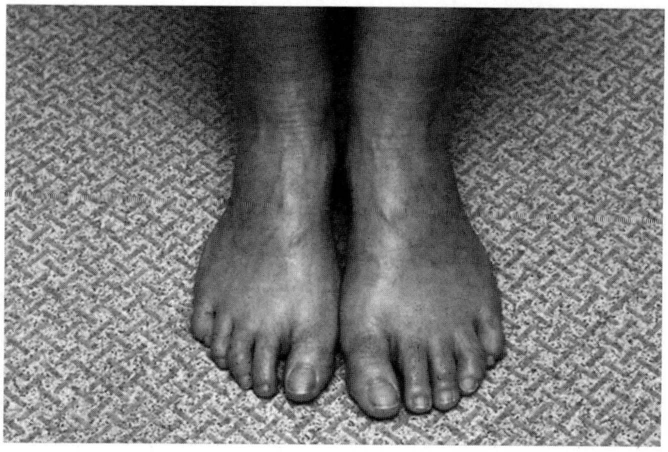

FIGURE 79–4 Asymmetric feet of a diastematomyelia patient.

pelvic floor. Congenital scoliosis is another form of presentation.

The diagnosis can be made by viewing a computed tomography (CT) myelogram or MRI. Sometimes abnormal segmentation or the median septum can be seen on x-ray. Scoliosis and progressive neurologic deficit are surgical indications. In addition, children with diastematomyelia should be considered for surgery because they are at risk for neurologic damage during growth spurts secondary to cord tethering. Adults with new-onset bladder or other neurologic symptoms are surgical candidates and are often diagnosed after a seemingly minor trauma.

Utilizing microsurgical technique and electrophysiologic monitoring, the median septum should be fully resected, and the two dural sacs (if present) should be converted to one sac. Because the cord is tethered caudally, removal of the septum is cephalad to caudad, to minimize trauma to the cord. Conscientious hemostasis should be practiced at the septum/vertebral body interface, as well as the epidural space; these will be sources of bleeding. Dural closure will require a dural patch graft.

SUGGESTED READING

Sami H, Ross E, Walter M, Goli S. Split spinal cord (diastematomyelia). Neurology 2003;60:491

80

Spinal Teratoma

■ Presentation

A 38-year-old woman had urinary retention. Workup found a large sacral teratoma, and she underwent a subtotal resection, with some clinical improvement. She had further medical treatment and pain management, but currently presents with worsening urinary symptoms and mild right lower extremity weakness.

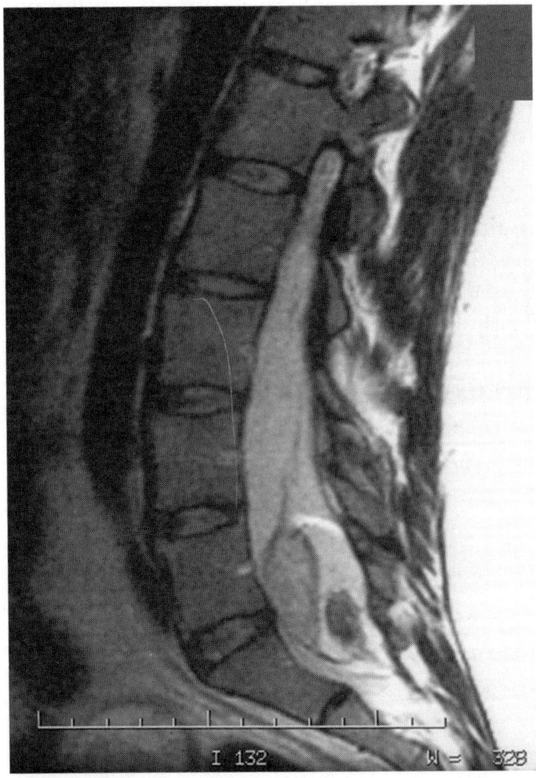

FIGURE 80–1 Sagittal view lumbosacral MRI shows a heterogenous intradural, tethering lesion.

■ Radiologic Findings

Recurrent teratoma is seen behind the L5–S1 segment on magnetic resonance imaging (MRI) (**Figs. 80–1** and **80–2**). A heterogeneous intradural lesion is observed tethering the spinal cord down to L5. Spina bifida is also noted.

■ Pathology Findings and Diagnosis

Recurrent teratoma. Specimen from the filum terminale is described as adipose tissue (**Fig. 80–3**). Specimen from the intradural mass is diagnosed as a mature teratoma with cuboidal and squamous elements and mature sebaceous sweat glands (**Fig. 80–4**).

■ Treatment

This patient had a redo lumbosacral laminectomy, adhesiolysis, and tethered cord release.

■ Discussion

This patient has a chronic cauda equina–type picture, with a recurrent, hard to treat lesion. Gross total surgical resection is recommended at the onset, because further surgical attempts carry a significant morbidity and are very challenging. In this case, her tethered cord must be released with lysis of adhesions, to alleviate her symptoms.

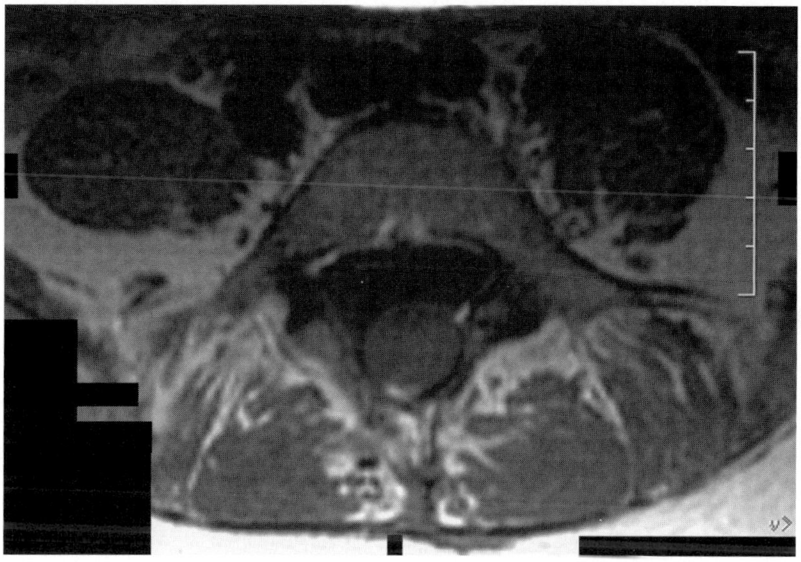

FIGURE 80–2 Axial lumbosacral MRI gives a different view of this teratoma.

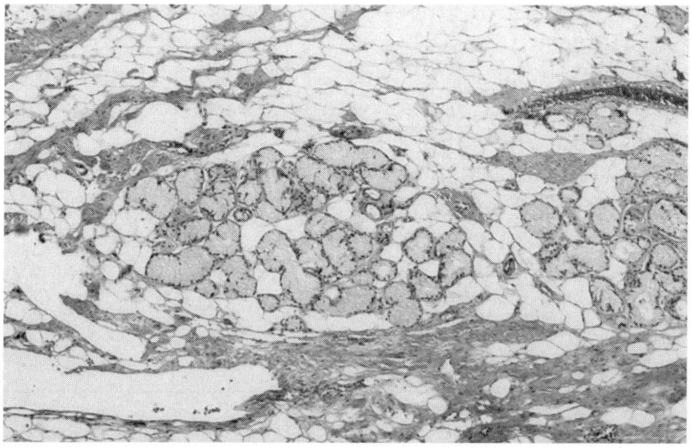

FIGURE 80–3 Specimen from the filum terminale is described as adipose tissue.

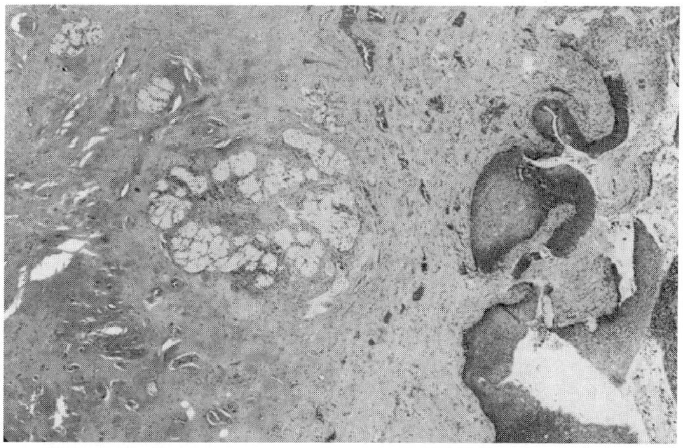

FIGURE 80–4 Specimen from the intradural mass is diagnosed as a mature teratoma with cuboidal and squamous elements and mature sebaceous sweat glands.

Such procedures must be done using precise microsurgical technique, nerve root monitoring intraoperatively, and preoperative nerve conduction studies of the L5, S1, and bladder and sphincter roots for baseline.

SUGGESTED READING

Sharma MC, Aggarwal M, Ralte AM, et al. Clinicopathological study of spinal teratomas. A series of 10 cases. J Neurosurg Sci 2003;47: 95–100

81

Congenital Abnormality of the Spine

▪ Presentation

A 41-year-old woman with known congenital abnormalities of the spine complained of lower extremity radiculopathy. She had decreased left S1 sensation and a tuft of hair overlaying the thoracolumbar junction.

▪ Radiologic Findings

Magnetic resonance imaging (MRI) of the whole spine was reviewed, and it is notable for numerous pathologies. In addition to segmentation anomalies and spondylolysis, there are several intradural findings. The T2-weighted sagittal MRI of the thoracic spine shows intramedullary hyperintensity (**Fig. 81–1**). The same sequence shows a scoliotic lumbar spine, with grade II L5–S1 spondylolisthesis and a large heterogenous lesion displacing the cauda equina (**Fig. 81–2**). There is also diastematomyelia type II (**Figs. 81–3** and **81–4**) that extends from the lumbar to thoracic spine. The diastematomyelia tapers into a common thecal sac above and below the spur, as noted in the myelogram (**Fig. 81–5**).

▪ Diagnosis

Spina bifida occulta, with diastematomyelia, tethered cord, teratoma, and spondylolisthesis

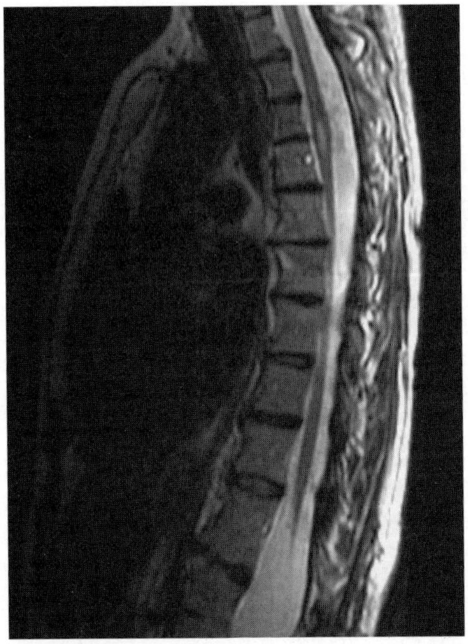

FIGURE 81–1 MRI showing a thoracic intramedullary lesion with a syrinx.

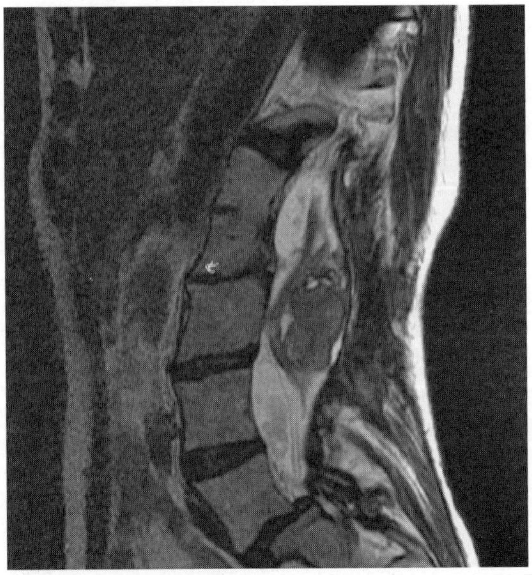

FIGURE 81–2 MRI demonstrating a large heterogenous intradural lumbar lesion.

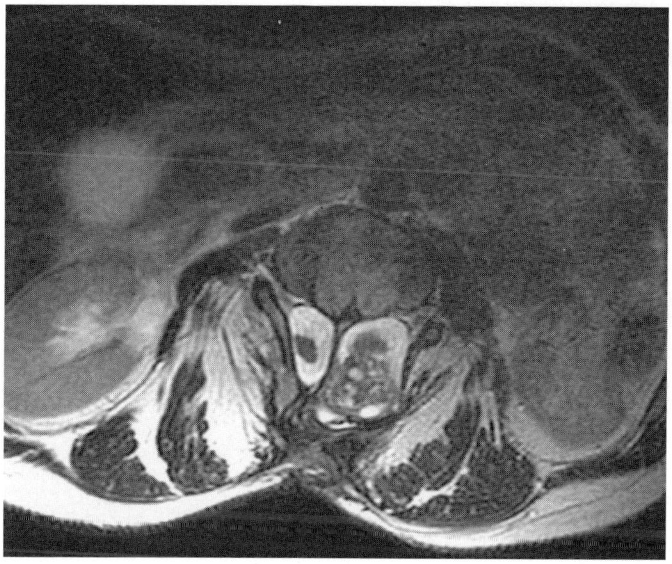

FIGURE 81–3 Axial MRI through the area with diastematomyelia and teratoma.

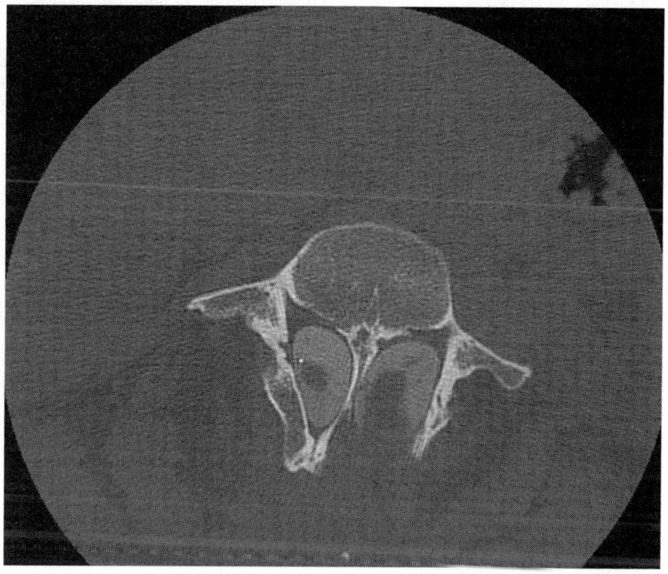

FIGURE 81–4 CT myelogram displaying the split cord malformation.

■ Treatment

The patient underwent a microsurgical tumor resection in conjunction with a diastematomyelia septal resection and cord untethering.

■ Discussion

This case is a fascinating constellation of congenital abnormalities. The patient has a type II diastematomyelia from T3 to L5, with cord tethering from a teratoma. There is a satellite intramedullary thoracic lesion with a syrinx, and multilevel thoracic vertebral segmentation abnormalities. L5 has a spondylolysis as well as a grade II L5–S1 spondylolisthesis. The combination of these pathologies has resulted in congenital scoliosis with a primary thoracic dextrocurvature and a secondary lumbar levocurvature.

Patients with these congenital abnormalities should undergo preoperative testing that includes urodynamic studies, and documentation of myelopathy or sensory deficits. The progression of this patient's intradural lesions and scoliosis should be assessed by reviewing previous studies. The lumbar tumor should be surgically treated, but the thoracic intramedullary lesion and syrinx can be serially scanned until they become symptomatic or significantly radiologically progressive. The decision was made to delay correction of her scoliosis and first address the lumbar lesion and diastematomyelia. Tethering is the first problem to address. Once the patient recovers from treatment of these underlying tethering lesions, a longer fusion surgery can be planned. On the other hand, some surgeons may prefer to accomplish the microsurgical work and fusion in one setting to avoid the comorbidities associated with further reoperation. Both options are viable alternatives in the treatment of this multifaceted and complicated case.

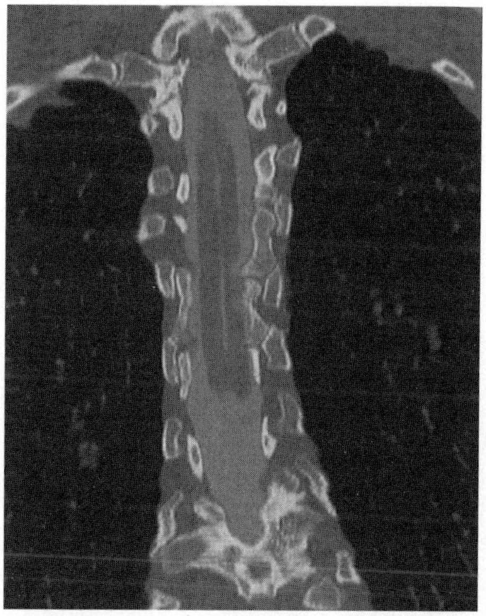

FIGURE 81–5 CT myelogram notable for the thoracic extent of the split cord malformation.

SUGGESTED READING

Hader WJ, Steinbok P, Poskitt K, Hendson G. Intramedullary spinal teratoma and distematomyelia. Case report and review of the literature. Pediatr Neurosurg 1999;30:140–145

82

Thoracic Arteriovenous Fistula

■ Presentation

A 75-year-old man complained of increasing difficulty walking. He had a sensory level at T10–T11.

■ Radiologic Findings

T2-weighted thoracic magnetic resonance imaging (MRI) (**Fig. 82–1**) showed multiple flow voids in the dorsal aspect of the thoracic canal. A myelogram (**Fig. 82–2**) revealed a thoracic block with the presence of serpentine vessels.

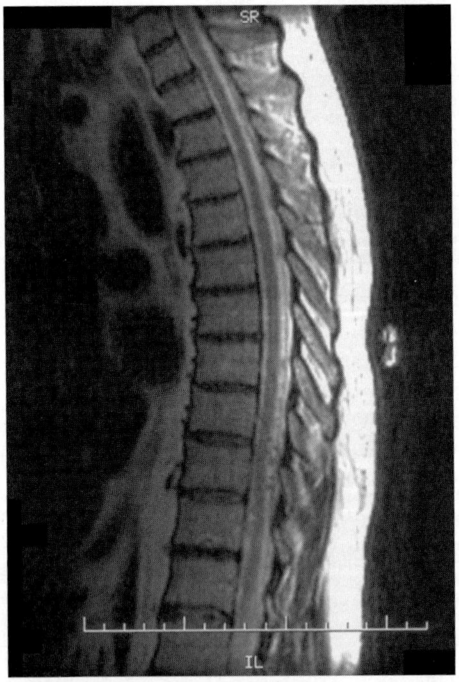

FIGURE 82–1 MRI with multiple flow voids seen in the dorsal aspect of the thoracic canal.

A spinal angiogram (**Fig. 82–3**) showed a lower thoracic arteriovenous fistula with a feeding artery stemming from a right T7 radial artery. The artery of Adamkiewicz was identified on the left at T12.

■ Diagnosis

Type I spinal arteriovenous fistula

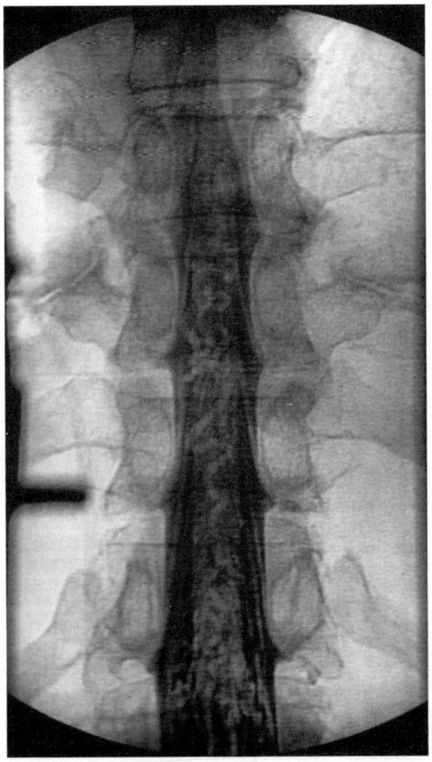

FIGURE 82–2 Serpentine vessels seen on myelogram.

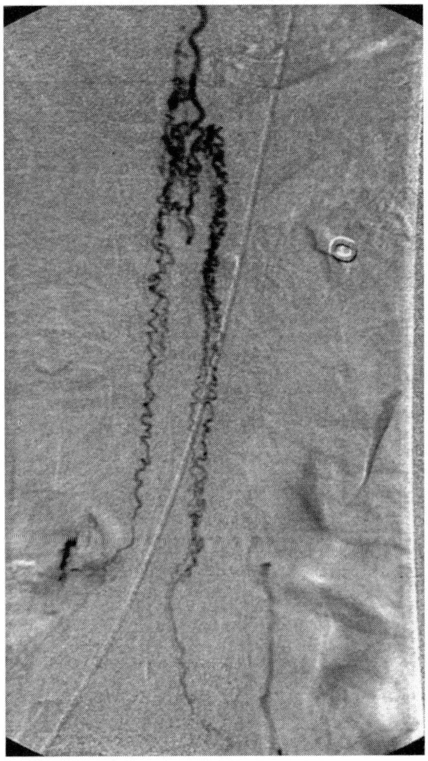

FIGURE 82–3 Spinal angiogram with radial artery feeding vessel.

■ Treatment

A T6–T8 laminectomy with durotomy was completed. At the T7 level, a large arterialized vein was seen piercing the dura and connecting with serpentine veins of the spinal cord. These veins were dilated and arterialized. The feeding artery was clipped at its entrance to the dura. Six weeks after surgery the patient had regained leg strength and was able to walk 2 miles.

■ Discussion

There are four types of spinal arteriovenous malformations (AVMs). Type I is a dural AVM, fed by a dural artery and draining into a spinal vein in the foramen. This type is best treated surgically. Type II is an intradural extramedullary AVM that also responds well to surgery. Type III is intramedullary, and can respond to embolization. This type has the worst prognosis. Finally, type IV is a perimedullary AVM that can be treated surgically or interventionally, depending on the arterial supply and venous drainage.

There are two treatment options for spinal arteriovenous fistulas. One treatment option is through embolization of the draining vein. This treatment can cause a cord infarct. The patient will have to undergo follow-up spinal angiograms, and may end up needing surgery if the embolization is ultimately unsuccessful. Surgery is the alternative and involves disconnecting the arteriovenous pedicle.

SUGGESTED READING

Song JK, Vinuela F, Gobin YP, et al. Surgical and endovascular treatment of spinal dural arteriovenous fistulas: long-term disability assessment and prognostic factors. J Neurosurg 2001;94:199–204

83

Arachnoid Cyst

▪ Presentation

A 60-year-old man who had a previous thoracic laminectomy for resection of an arachnoid cyst continued to have progressive myelopathy.

▪ Radiologic Findings

T2-weighted sagittal magnetic resonance imaging (MRI) of the spine shows a septated arachnoid cyst spanning from the cervicomedullary junction into the thoracic spine (**Figs. 83–1** and **83–2**). The cyst is cerebrospinal fluid (CSF) density on MRI. The individual compartments communicate as seen on myelogram (**Figs. 83–3** and **83–4**).

▪ Diagnosis

Recurrent, enlarging, spinal arachnoid cyst

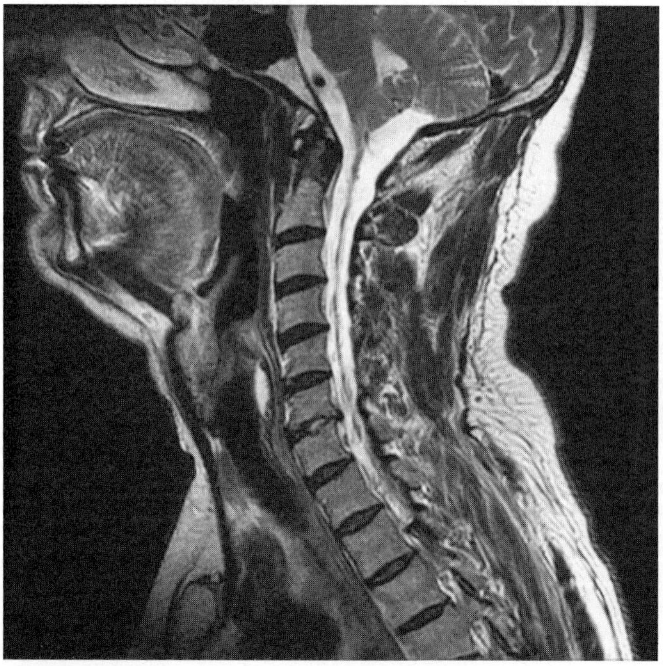

FIGURE 83–1 MRI of the cervical spine demonstrates the arachnoid cyst.

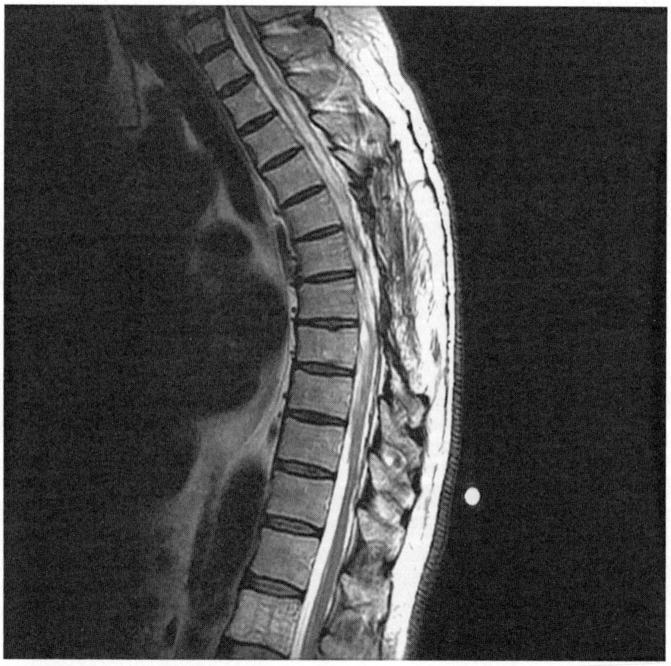

FIGURE 83–2 MRI of the thoracic spine demonstrates the arachnoid cyst.

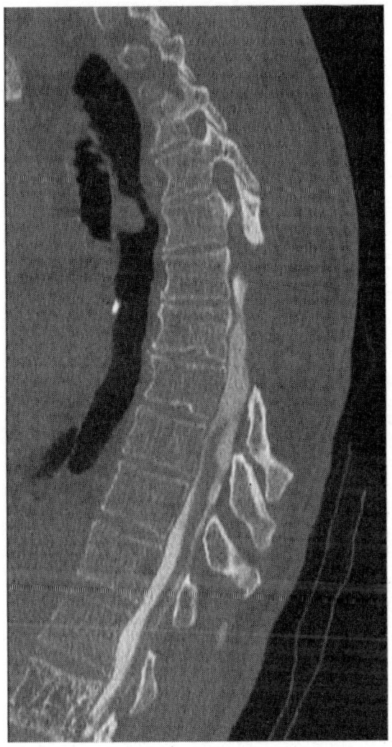

FIGURE 83–3 Communication within the cyst is seen on myelogram.

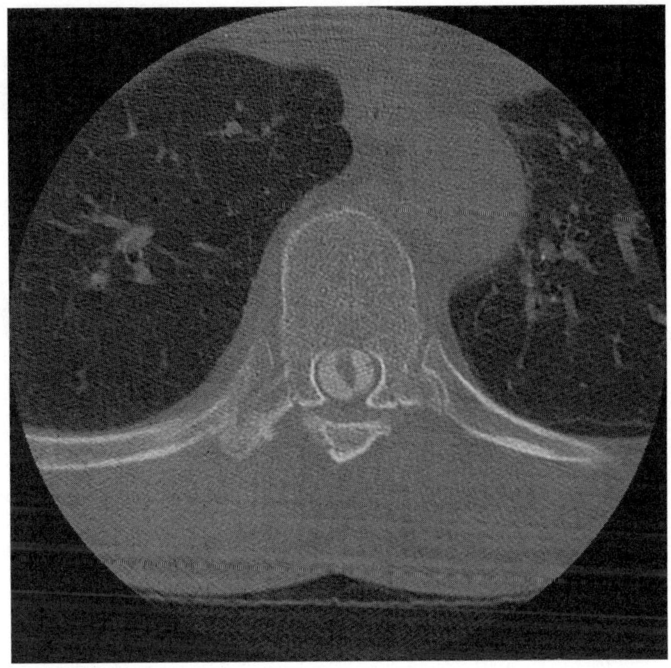

FIGURE 83–4 Axial CT myelogram slice through the arachnoid cyst.

■ Treatment

A thoracic laminectomy for lysis of arachnoiditis adhesions and placement of a syringopleural shunt was done.

■ Discussion

Arachnoid cysts contain CSF and are intra-arachnoid in location. They can occur in the brain or spine. In the spine they are usually dorsal to the thoracic cord, and result from a congenital defect or from previous trauma, surgery, or infection. Arachnoid cysts are created when the arachnoid membrane splits, forming a cyst cavity that is devoid of vasculature. They can expand when pulse waves of CSF become entrapped in the arachnoid, and may be unilocular or septated.

Arachnoid cysts may be associated with scoliosis or spinal dysraphism; however, patients with these cysts are often asymptomatic and discover them by accident. MRI and computed tomography (CT) myelography are the tests of choice, and the latter can demonstrate if communication exists within a septated cyst. If the spinal canal is widened enough, pedicle erosion can occur. Symptoms depend on location. The spinal differential includes meningocele, dorsal nerve root ganglia cysts, extradural ganglion cysts, and Tarlov cysts.

Treatment of asymptomatic patients is debatable, with most authors advocating no intervention. If a spinal arachnoid cyst is symptomatic, the cyst's outer membrane should be excised and then the fluid shunted, usually to the pleural or peritoneal space. If no shunting is done, the membranes may not remain fenestrated. In this patient's case, although myelopathy is often progressive, investigation for repairable causes is still necessary. In addition, his previous surgery with arachnoiditis puts him at risk for further cyst development.

SUGGESTED READING

Cakirer S. Arachnoid cyst of the craniospinal junction: a case report and review of the literature. Acta Radiol 2004;45:460–463

84

Achondroplasia

■ Presentation

A 46-year-old achondroplastic dwarf came to the emergency department with cauda equina syndrome.

■ Radiologic Findings

A sagittal view, reconstructed computed tomography (CT) myelogram of the lumbar spine is seen, notable for the dysmorphic vertebral bodies and severe congenital spinal canal stenosis seen in this disorder (**Fig. 84–1**).

■ Diagnosis

Spinal stenosis in an achondroplastic dwarf

■ Treatment

An emergent lumbar laminectomy was done.

■ Discussion

There are hundreds of types of dwarfism, and achondroplasia is the most common. Achondroplastic dwarfs have short arms and legs, an enlarged head, and an average size trunk. They are about 4 feet in height. Abnormal endochondral ossification is the primary defect. This disorder has an autosomal-dominant inheritance, but ~80% of cases are due to a new mutation. Intelligence is normal. The most common health problems faced by this population are craniovertebral junction anomalies, lumbar stenosis, otitis media, sleep apnea, and obesity.

The spine in achondroplastic children prior to ambulation has a thoracolumbar kyphosis, but corrects to an exaggerated lumbar lordosis with the development of ambulation. This spinal deformity is associated with hip flexion contractures and genu varum. Spinal stenosis can be severe in these patients. The pedicles and laminae

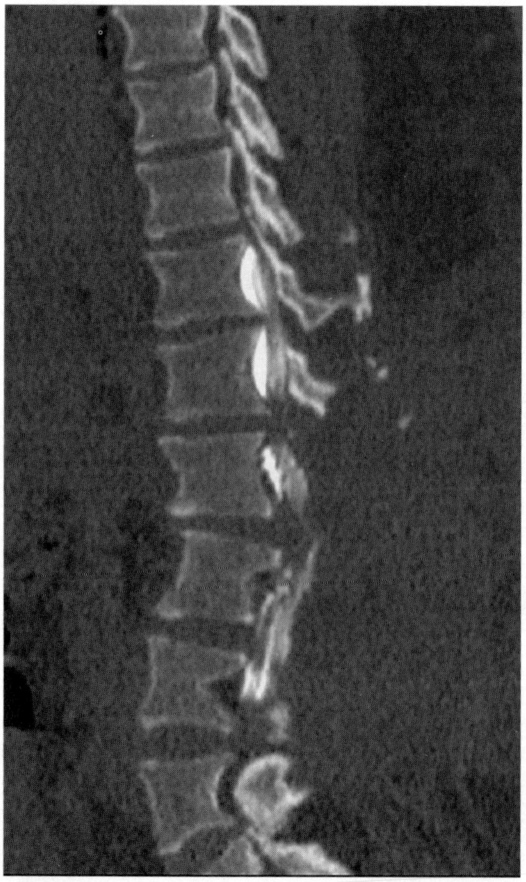

FIGURE 84–1 Severe canal stenosis is noted on this CT myelogram of the thoracolumbar spine.

are short and thick, and there is interpedicular narrowing, associated disc herniations, and vertebral body wedging.

Children diagnosed with achondroplasia should be genetically tested. Cranial and spinal imaging should be obtained, with special attention to the craniovertebral junction. Potential morbidity can be averted if cervicomedullary compression at the foramen magnum, hydrocephalus, atlantoaxial abnormalities, or subaxial stenosis is diagnosed prior to the development of a fixed deficit.

Spinal procedures are usually decompressive, whether at the C0–C1 junction or caudally. Laminectomies should be wide and multilevel, with attention to the lateral recesses to be successful. Fusion may be necessary to prevent postlaminectomy instability. Additionally, thoracolumbar kyphosis over 30 degrees, persisting after independent ambulation, should be corrected. The congenitally narrow canal warrants special consideration during instrumentation. Hooks and claws are contraindicated as they will additionally stenose the canal. Often, a decompression and anterior-posterior fusion is necessary for safe deformity correction.

SUGGESTED READING

Bethem D, Winter RB, Lutter L, et al. Spinal disorders of dwarfism. Review of the literature and report of eighty cases. J Bone Joint Surg Am 1981;63:1412–1425

85

Arachnoiditis

■ Presentation

An 87-year-old woman presented with chronic low back pain radiating to the posterior thighs. She had two lumbar decompressions and one non-instrumented fusion in the past. In addition, she has had several oil-based myelograms throughout her life. She is neurologically normal.

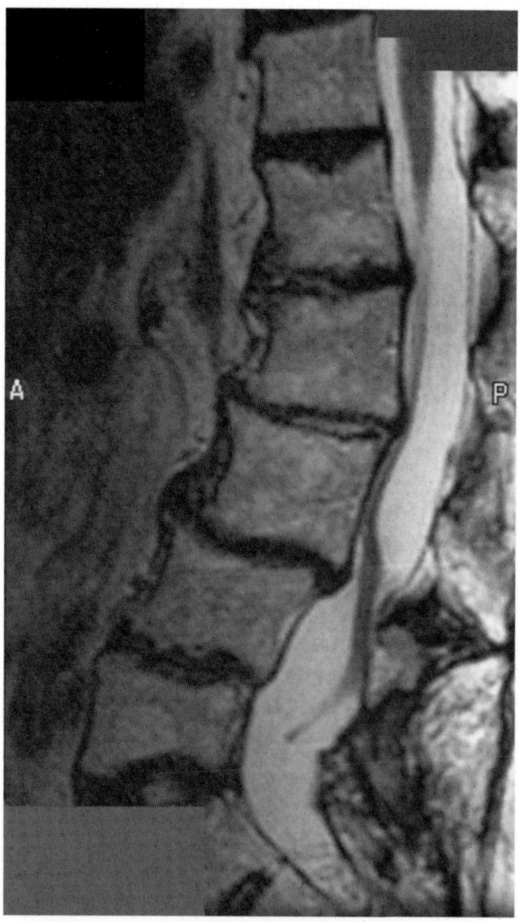

FIGURE 85–1 Sagittal MRI of the lumbar spine shows clumping of the cauda equina.

■ Radiologic Findings

Sagittal and axial T2-weighted magnetic resonance imaging (MRI) of the lumbar spine highlights spondylotic as well as postoperative changes, with notable nerve root clumping (**Figs. 85–1** and **85–2**).

■ Diagnosis

Arachnoiditis

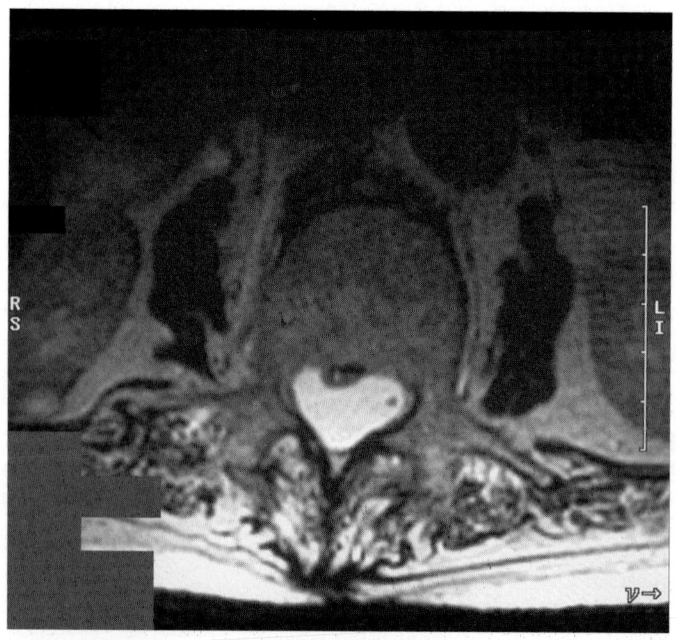

FIGURE 85–2 Axial MRI of the lumbar spine shows the same grouping of nerve roots.

■ Treatment

Pain management

■ Discussion

This patient's MRI shows a classic picture of nerve root clumping and an empty thecal sac, as found in arachnoiditis, which is an irritation of the nerve roots. It is likely that her multiple oil-based myelograms, from the 1970s onward, are the cause. Unfortunately, there is no surgical solution for arachnoiditis. These patients are best managed by referral to a pain clinic, and therapy to optimize physical conditioning.

SUGGESTED READING

Wright MH, Denney LC. A comprehensive review of spinal arachnoiditis. Orthop Nurs 2003;22:215–219

86

Spinal Deformity

■ Presentation

A 40-year-old woman with a history of back pain since adolescence complained of worsening pain but no neurologic deficit.

■ Radiologic Findings

Reconstructed computed tomography (CT) scan of the cervicothoracic spine is notable for extreme thoracic kyphosis and vertebral segmentation anomaly (**Fig. 86–1**).

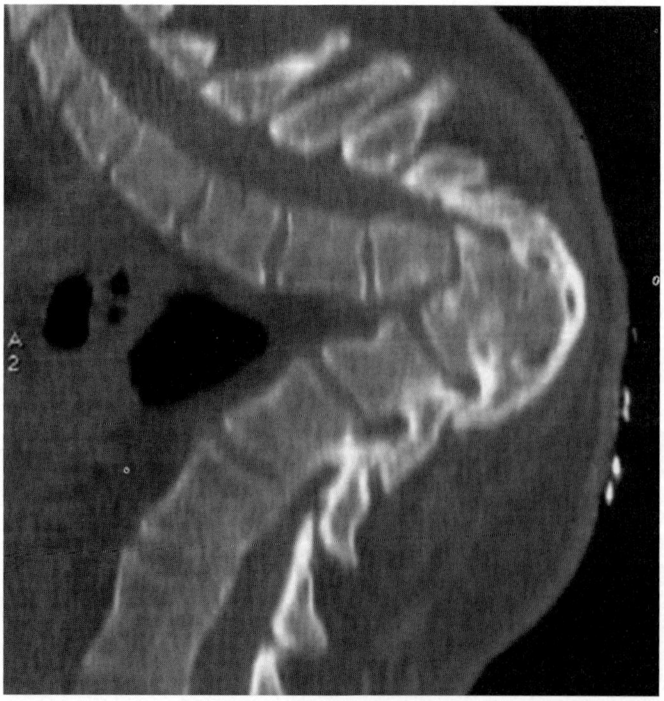

FIGURE 86–1 Dramatic thoracic kyphosis with segmentation anomaly.

■ Diagnosis

Congenital kyphotic deformity of the spine

■ Treatment

Surgical deformity correction

■ Discussion

Congenital kyphotic deformity of the spine encompasses a variety of spinal anomalies. Scoliosis with kyphosis or lordosis results from formation or segmentation failure. Failures of formation are hemivertebra and wedge vertebra, and segmentation failures include unilateral unsegmented bar and block vertebra. Over 50% of these patients have additional anomalies that can be related to the neuraxis (tethered cord, syringomyelia, or most commonly diastematomyelia), or related to other organs (musculoskeletal, genitourinary, or cardiovascular). Screening tests to look for associated abnormalities are strongly recommended and routine procedure prior to any surgical correction of these deformities.

Congenital kyphotic deformities almost always involve the thoracic and thoracolumbar spine. Neurologic findings are more common if kyphosis has resulted from failure of formation. This produces a sharp angular gibbus compared with the smooth, round kyphosis seen in failure of segmentation.

The presence of neurologic findings, curve progression, and patient age at time of presentation dictate treatment options. Children with kyphosis secondary to failure of formation are fused posteriorly in situ if there is less than 55 degrees of angulation. Additional anterior releases are necessary if the kyphosis is 55 degrees or greater.

Attempting to correct a severe kyphosis carries a high risk of neurologic deficit.

In the older patient with a milder deformity, particularly when related to segmentation failure, posterior fixation is adequate. The extracavitary approach can be used for patients with more dramatic corrective needs (e.g., decompression, vertebral osteotomy, and strut grafting), followed by posterior multilevel segmental fusion.

SUGGESTED READING

Winter RB, Moe HH, Wang JF. Congenital kyphosis: its natural history and treatment as observed in a study of one hundred and thirty patients. J Bone Joint Surg Am 1973;55:223–256

87

Tethered Cord

■ Presentation

A 31-year-old woman reported persistent back pain a few weeks after childbirth. She had some urinary retention, lower extremity dysesthesias, and had a long-standing tuft of hair on her lower back (**Fig. 87–1**).

■ Radiologic Findings

A T2-weighted sagittal lumbar magnetic resonance imaging (MRI) is remarkable for a low-lying conus (**Fig. 87–2**).

■ Diagnosis

Occult spinal dysraphism

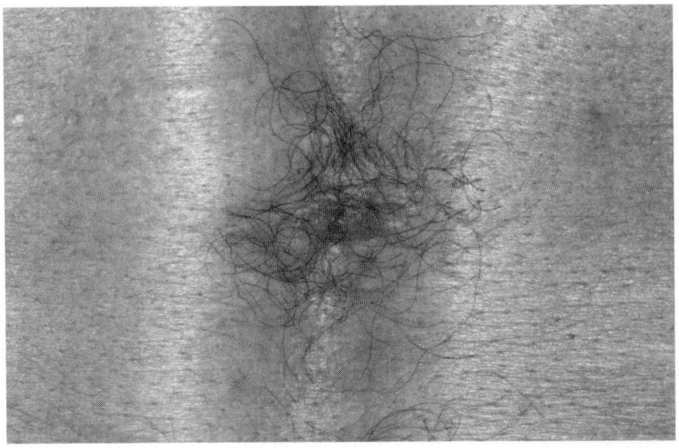

FIGURE 87–1 This tuft of hair was found on the patient's low back.

■ Treatment

A surgical de-tethering was accomplished, using neurophysiologic monitoring and microsurgical technique.

■ Discussion

The concept of spinal cord tethering has evolved to represent a gamut of congenital spinal dysraphic anomalies with a low-lying conus. In tethered cord, the conus lies

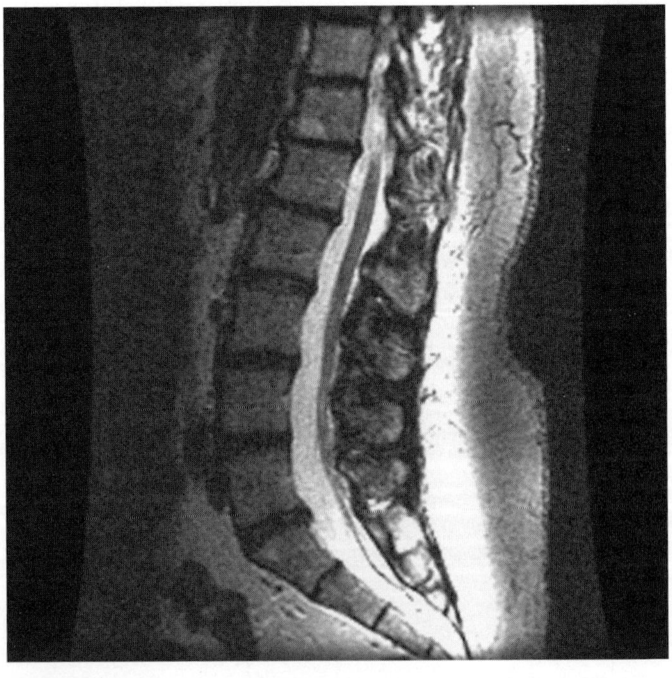

FIGURE 87–2 Lumbar MRI with a low-lying conus.

below the L1 vertebral body, and the patient may or may not have neurologic deficit. The cord can be tethered primarily from a thickened filum terminale or in association with other tethering pathologies, such as a lipoma, diastematomyelia, dermal sinus tract, or myelomeningocele, and can also be iatrogenic after repair of one of the aforementioned abnormalities. Also, there have been case reports of patients who present with clinical symptoms of tethered cord with the conus above the border of the L1 vertebral body.

The clinical presentation of tethered cord can take different forms, some similar to the presentation of diastematomyelia. Orthopedic foot and limb deformity, scoliosis, neurologic deficit, cutaneous marking, and an incidental radiologic finding after a seemingly unrelated incident are some examples. As in this case, the lithotomy position can be a trigger. Treatment is directed at the underlying pathology (i.e., lipoma resection, myelomeningocele repair, median septum resection in split cord malformation) to achieve cord untethering. Tandem lesions can be seen in up to 15% of cases. Imaging of the whole neuraxis is strongly recommended preoperatively.

Microsurgical technique and intraoperative neurophysiologic monitoring can help attain a successful outcome, and are essential to these cases. These lesions should be treated early and prior to the onset of neurologic symptoms, particularly in younger patients. Often the neurologic deficit is not reversible.

SUGGESTED READING

Krassioukov AV, Sarjeant R, Arkia H, Fehlings MG. Multimodality intraoperative monitoring during complex lumbosacral procedures: indications, techniques, and long-term follow-up review of 61 consecutive cases. J Neurosurg Spine 2004;1:243–253

Index

T

V

W